Lung Disease 101:

A Patient Primer

Arunabh Talwar, M.D., F.C.C.P.

Editorial Assistance

Sonu Sahni, M.D.

With Contributions From

Sam Davidoff, M.D.
Jose Cardenas-Garcia, M.D.
Donna Tsang, R.R.T.

Disclaimer

This book is not intended to replace a physician's advice. While medical professionals are writing this book, there is no substitute for personalized medical care. Every person has individual needs and not every statement in this book will apply to your personal health. You should consult your doctor before making any changes in your healthcare or following any advice you may find in this book.

Table of Contents

Chapter 1

Breathing Basics

"Breath is the bridge which connects life to consciousness, which unites your body to your thoughts."

Thich Nhat Hanh (b. 1926)

Let's first review the basic mechanisms and anatomical components of breathing. The main function of the lungs are to help us inhale air, transfer oxygen to our blood and help remove carbon dioxide from our body.

Anatomical Structures of the Lung

Upper Airways
Includes the nose, mouth and throat. Air is warmed, filtered and humidified by these structures as it passes through the upper airways.

Trachea
A tube-like structure allowing air to pass between the throat and the lung, also known as the windpipe.

Bronchi
Two main branches of the trachea leading to the left and right lungs. Bronchi further subdivide in the lungs forming a bronchial tree.

Bronchiole
Smaller branches of bronchi.

Alveoli
Sac like structures at the end of the bronchioles. They are thin walled allowing for the exchange of oxygen and carbon dioxide between the lungs and the bloodstream.

Interstitium
Area between two alveoli where tiny blood vessels (capillaries) are located.

Mucous Membrane
A thin membrane lining the breathing passages beginning at the nose and ending in the small bronchi covered with mucous producing glands. Mucus is a slimy substance that airways produce to help remove inhaled dust, bacteria and other small particles.

Diaphragm
A large muscle dividing the abdominal cavity and chest that is the main muscle of breathing.

The primary function of the lung is to transfer oxygen from the air into the body and to remove carbon dioxide. Oxygen acts as the body's fuel, while carbon dioxide is a waste product. Air enters the lungs through the upper airways eventually reaching the air sacs (alveoli). The alveoli are surrounded by many tiny blood vessels known as capillaries. It is here, at the meeting point between blood vessels and alveoli that blood is oxygenated and carbon dioxide is released and exhaled.

The normal lung has a mechanism for defending itself against foreign particles. Mucous glands and little hair-like structures, known as cilia are found in the walls lining the bronchial tubes. Whenever a foreign particle enters the lung it is trapped by a blanket of mucous and wave-like motions of the cilia move it up and away from the lung to the mouth where it is exhaled by coughing.

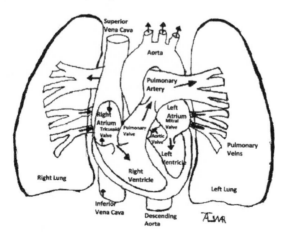

Chapter 2

Diseases of the Lung

"I claim that in losing the spinning wheel we lost our left lung. We are, therefore, suffering from galloping consumption. The restoration of the wheel arrests the progress of the fell disease."

Mahatma Gandhi (1869-1948)

There are many existing lung diseases. Let us review a few common lung diseases that result in chronic illness. All chronic lung diseases, if not treated, result in progressive shortness of breath (SOB). Below you will find a few examples of lung disease.

Table 1: Common examples of Lung Diseases

Diseases of Upper Airways	Infection of the sinuses, tonsils
Diseases of Lower Airways	Diseases involving trachea, bronchi and bronchioles, Chronic obstructive pulmonary disease (COPD), Asthma, Bronchiectasis (inflammation and dilatation of airways)
Pulmonary Artery	Pulmonary Arterial Hypertension, Pulmonary Embolism.
Pleura	Pleural effusion - fluid buildup in the pleura - a structure around the lung
Alveoli	Pneumonia, Viral Flu
Interstitium	Interstitial lung diseases

Chronic Obstructive Pulmonary Disease (COPD)

Chronic obstructive pulmonary disease (COPD) refers to a condition of the lungs that makes breathing more difficult.

In this condition the airways are either narrowed by inflammation or a spasm of the airways (bronchospasm). When an individual breathes in the chest expands creating a vacuum that draws air into the lungs and causes the airways to open. During expiration, the chest volume decreases and the airways (already narrow) collapse and trap the air in the alveoli. And so air enters more freely than it exits and the residual volume of the lungs (contained trapped air) increases. Vital capacity (maximum amount of air a person can expel from the lungs after a maximum inhalation) decreases. Fresh incoming air from the next inspiration mixes with the retained air. This leads to a decrease in the concentration of oxygen in the alveoli and to a decrease in the oxygen delivered to the tissues.

COPD is a progressive condition that is characteristically not fully reversible. However, if you get appropriate treatment and make lifestyle changes, you can slow the damage and improve your lung function which will help you cough less, breathe more efficiently and feel better.

Chronic = always present to some degree
Obstructive = blockage in the airways
Pulmonary = lungs
Disease = illness

The most common syndromes are chronic bronchitis and emphysema. Please note that these are often found in combination, so a patient diagnosed with COPD can have both emphysema and bronchitis, simultaneously.

Chronic Bronchitis

This lung disease causes inflammation in the airways and overproduction of mucus. Inflammation narrowing and mucous plugging can clog the airways, making it difficult to breathe. Excess mucus is a common feature of this disease. Chronic bronchitis occurs as a result of constant irritation of the airways from cigarette smoke or other inhaled substances. A constant cough develops in an attempt to rid the lungs of the excess mucus. Although we all cough, chronic bronchitis patients have a cough with excessive mucous which occurs for at least three months out of a year for two consecutive years.

Emphysema

Worldwide, cigarette smoking is the most overwhelmingly common cause for emphysema. Other exposures which can cause emphysema include occupational dusts and indoor air pollution from biomass fuel used for cooking. In addition, any factor that affects lung growth prior to birth and during childhood (low birth weight, respiratory infections, etc.) has the potential for increasing an individual's chances of developing emphysema. Whereas chronic bronchitis is a disease of the airways, emphysema is a disease of the air sacs, or alveoli.

Emphysema causes inflammation and damage to the fragile walls of the air sacs in the deepest part of the lungs. This structural damage causes the air sacs and small airways of your lungs to collapse as you breathe out. Constant irritation from smoke or other pollutants damage the airways causing them to become narrow and thereby limiting the passage of air leaving the lungs. As a result air becomes trapped inside the alveoli causing them to distend and eventually rupture. These damaged alveoli, provide less surface area for the exchange of oxygen and carbon dioxide resulting in a less efficient way of breathing.

Another rare cause of emphysema is related to a genetic condition causing deficiency of a particular lung repair enzyme which occurs in only 0.03% of the US population. Alpha-1 proteinase inhibitor or Alpha-1 antitrypsin (AAT) deficiency is a genetic or inherited disorder caused by a lack of AAT which is produced mostly in the liver. This enzyme allows for maintenance of proper elasticity of the lungs and prevents lung degradation. Though the mechanism differs from smoking related emphysema, the end result and symptomology are the same. Treatment is focused on early detection and slowing the progression with bronchodilators inhalers and antibiotics. If you develop lung infections, doctors may prescribe AAT replacement or augmentation therapy.

What Are the Symptoms of COPD?

- Cough with mucous that doesn't go away.
- Shortness of breath or wheezing that may begin with exercise.
- You may feel short of breath during exercise, even walking at a casual pace or during simple, everyday activities.
- It may take longer to recover from lung infections.

It's possible to have COPD even if you're asymptomatic. Generally, more severe symptoms mean more lung damage. COPD patients are more prone to develop severe upper and lower respiratory tract infections or chronic respiratory failure. Your doctor can perform simple breathing tests to better gauge how severe your disease is.

What is the Treatment for COPD?

There are four main components in the therapy of COPD:

- Avoid smoking (refer to Chapter 10 – Lung and Tobacco)
- Maintain up to date vaccinations (influenza and pneumococcal)
- Long term medications - long term controllers which include steroids and anti-cholinergics (refer to Chapter 4 – Pulmonary Medications). The controller medications are used over a period of time to minimize symptoms on a daily basis.
- Pulmonary rehabilitation.
- In rare cases, surgical intervention may be needed; your physician will discuss this further as an option.

Asthma

Asthma is a chronic lung disease that causes episodes of chest tightness, wheezing and shortness of breath. Approximately 34 million people in the United States suffer from wheezing and discomfort caused by asthma. The symptoms are primarily due to tightening of muscles surrounding the airways, inflammation and irritation of the airways in the lungs.

What are the Causes of Asthma?

Incidence of asthma has increased dramatically over the last several decades. While the exact cause of asthma is still unknown, many think the following factors may contribute to the development of asthma:
- Atopy, or an inherited tendency to develop allergies
- Family history of asthma or allergy.
- Contracting certain viral respiratory infections in early childhood.
- Exposure to some airborne allergens (pollens, smoke, pet dander, etc.) and other allergens like dust mites or indoor molds.

- Hyperreactive airways (exaggerated airway response to stimuli)

Asthma symptoms wax and wane over time, with treatment focused on prevention, control and reducing airway reactivity and airway inflammation.

What are the Symptoms of Asthma?

The constriction and inflammation may cause patients to experience some or all of the following classical symptoms of asthma:

- Wheezing
- Chest tightness
- Shortness of breath
- Chronic cough

All cases of asthma are different and individuals may exhibit different symptoms. Some of the common types of asthma are as follows:

Allergic (Extrinsic) Asthma - The most common types of Asthma; this is triggered by reaction to environmental allergens. Common ones are pollen, ragweed, pet dander and cigarette smoke.

Cough Variant Asthma – Such individuals experience a dry or non productive cough instead of wheezing or tightness in the chest.

Exercise Induced Asthma - Such individuals experience symptoms before or after periods of exercise or exertion.

Nocturnal Asthma - The symptoms occur between 10 p.m. and 2 a.m. Symptoms typically prevent sleep and are the result of a hormone dip, which interrupts body's natural sleep rhythm.

Occupational Asthma - In this condition the symptoms are a result of exposure to triggers in work place. Commonly seen amongst animal breeders, hairdressers, nurses, etc., the symptoms flare up while at work and decrease when they are away from workplace.

How is Asthma Diagnosed?

Diagnosing asthma requires 2 specific criteria, one of which is presence of symptoms compatible with asthma. In addition an objective measurement of decreased airflow in your lungs using a specific measurement like peak expiratory flow and measurements of patient's lung functions.

What is the Treatment for Asthma?

Treatment for your asthma will primarily involve three main components:

- Avoidance of triggers. The first step is recognizing the triggering factors and minimizing the exposure to such triggers. This is essential to control Asthma symptoms.
- Treatment with medications. Treatment falls into two categories: *long term controllers* and *rescue inhalers*. The controller medications are used over a period of time to minimize symptoms on a daily basis and reduce the chronic inflammation associated with asthma. Rescue inhalers are bronchodilators drugs that instantly improve the symptoms of wheezing. Rescue medications are those that are used specifically when asthma flares up causing an asthma attack. The controller medications can be in the form of inhalers or oral medicines. Of course even with daily controller medications you should always have a rescue inhaler with you to quickly relieve symptoms. In some patients treatment can be focused on preventing the body's immune response to allergy triggers. Physicians may use antibody injections to prevent allergy-associated asthma.
- Monitoring of your peak expiratory flow and asthma symptoms. Also beyond medications life style changes can be made to minimize the impact of asthma symptoms.

Bronchiectasis

Bronchiectasis is a condition in which damage to the airways causes them to widen and become flabby and scarred. It is usually the result of an infection, condition that injures the airways or prevents the airways from clearing mucus. When mucus can't be cleared, it builds up and creates an environment in which bacteria can grow which leads to recurring serious lung infections.

Each infection causes progressively increasing damage to your airways. Overtime, the airways lose their ability to move air in and out which can prevent adequate oxygenation of organs. Bronchiectasis can lead to serious health problems, such as respiratory failure, recurrent airway collapsing and pneumonia.

Management of Bronchiectasis

Bronchiectasis can't be cured; however with proper care quality of life is not affected. Early diagnosis and treatment of bronchiectasis are important. The underlying principle of therapy is to prevent further scarring and recurrent infection. Being up to date with influenza and pneumococcal vaccination is important. The sooner your doctor can start treating your bronchiectasis and any underlying associated medical conditions, the better the chances are of preventing further damage to your lungs.

Pneumonia

Pneumonia is a common lung infection caused by bacteria, virus or fungi. Pneumonia and its symptoms can vary from mild to severe. Most patients present with fever, chills, rigors and excessive tiredness. A chest X-ray is required to make a diagnosis.

The most common cause of bacterial pneumonia in adults is *Streptococcus pneumoniae* (pneumococcus), but there is a vaccine available for this form of pneumonia. There are other bacteria that can cause infection of the lungs that may have atypical features in presentation and are called atypical pneumonias, (also called walking pneumonia); this is caused by bacteria such as *Legionella pneumophila, Mycoplasma pneumoniae and Chlamydia pneumoniae.*

Patients require an antibiotic for treatment of pneumonia. Treatment depends on the cause of your pneumonia, how severe your symptoms are and your age and overall health. While most cases of pneumonia may be treated on an outpatient basis, severe cases require hospital admission. Most healthy people recover from pneumonia in one to three weeks, but pneumonia can be life threatening. The good news is that pneumonia can be prevented by getting an annual flu shot (as flu often leads to pneumonia), frequently washing your hands and for people at high risk, getting a vaccine for pneumococcal pneumonia.

The flu virus is the most common cause of viral pneumonia in adults. Other viruses that cause pneumonia include respiratory syncytial virus, rhinovirus, herpes simplex virus, severe acute respiratory syndrome (SARS) and more.

Cold or Flu

Influenza or flu is a viral infection that attacks the respiratory system: the nose, throat, bronchial tubes and lungs. Flu poses greatest risk to elderly adults, infants, those who have diabetes, chronic heart disease or lung disease or an impaired immune system. Although the intestinal ailments such as gastroenteritis, a condition that causes diarrhea, nausea and vomiting are often referred to as flu, they are not. It can be difficult to tell whether you have flu because many of the symptoms are similar to those of a common cold. A cold is a viral infection of the lung (mucus membrane) or the nose, throat and airways to the lungs. Flu (fever, chills, rigors, headache, fatigue) usually occur suddenly after an incubation of about one to four days. Flu symptoms last about a week. There are five tests available that your physician can use to diagnose flu as follows:

- Rapid screen for influenza A & B.
- Rapid screen for RSV (respiratory syncytial virus).
- Direct immunofluoresence test of sputum.
- Respiratory culture.
- Respiratory virus panel by polymerase chain reaction (PCR).

Rapid screen for influenza A & B viruses are used during the flu season, these test give results in short period of time, but they are not as sensitive or able to test for many different viruses as the other tests. In a suspected case of flu, a nasopharyngeal sample is sent for rapid screen. If that is negative then usually the sample is further tested by either viral culture or respiratory viral panel PCR. A culture can take 2-3 days to get an answer but a culture is more sensitive and can detect more types of viruses than the rapid tests. The respiratory viral panel by PCR is molecular test that uses PCR to amplify DNA or RNA from respiratory viruses present in the patient's nasopharyngeal swab or sputum sample. It is the most sensitive test and can detect up to 15 different viruses. Getting a yearly influenza vaccine (unless contraindicated) can greatly diminish your chances of getting the flu

Tuberculosis

Tuberculosis (TB) is a communicable infection (can be transmitted from person to person) that usually affects the lungs. It is spread by airborne droplets when an infected person coughs or sneezes. It is caused by a bacterium called *Mycobacterium tuberculosis*. There are two types of tuberculosis infections. One is dormant; know as latent tubercular infection (LTBI) and the other is active tuberculosis infection. At the time of diagnosis, people with active TB infection usually have a variety of symptoms such as low-grade fever, constant cough with sputum (phlegm), night sweats and unintentional weight loss.

Classifying TB

- Active TB describes an ongoing infection in which a person develops symptoms and has a positive (abnormal) result on a test for TB.
- Latent TB occurs when a person with no symptoms has a positive result on a TB skin or blood test. This suggests that the person was infected with TB in the past but the bacteria are in a dormant or inactive state. Persons with latent TB cannot spread the TB bacteria to others.
- Multidrug-resistant TB (MDR-TB) is a form of active TB caused by bacteria that do not respond to the medications most commonly used to treat TB.

Risk Factors for TB

- A deficient or weakened immune system, such as in people with diabetes or HIV/AIDS
- Traveling to or living in countries where tuberculosis is endemic (found commonly)
- Working in health care or refugee camps
- Living in overcrowded and poorly ventilated residences

Evaluation for suspected TB

- Tuberculin skin test (also called PPD or purified protein derivative). In response to this injection, if a person has been infected with TB, immune cells will indurate (harden) the area surrounding the injection site. The area of induration is measured 48 to 72 hours after injection and used to determine the likelihood of TB infection.

- Chest x-ray may be done to distinguish between active and latent TB.
- A blood test may be done to check for cytokines (substances released by immune cells) that are unique to TB infections. This test is called the QuntiFERON® TB Gold Test.

Treatment

- Several antimicrobials (medicines that kill microorganisms or interfere with their growth) are used to treat tuberculosis.
- Treatment usually lasts for 6 months and requires close monitoring by an infectious diseases specialist or other specialist.
- Complete treatment of a person with any form of TB is essential to maintain the person's health and to prevent the spread of tuberculosis to others.

Prevention

- In high-risk health care settings, appropriate precautions should be followed. This includes wearing masks specifically designed to prevent the spread of TB.
- Patients diagnosed as having latent TB may be given medications to kill dormant bacteria and prevent the development of active TB.
- In countries where TB is endemic, people may be given Bacille Calmette-Guerin (BCG), a vaccine against TB.

Pulmonary Embolism

A pulmonary embolism (PE) is a blood clot that blocks the blood vessels supplying the lungs. The clot (embolus) most often comes from the leg veins and travels through the heart to the lungs. When the blood clot lodges in the blood vessels of the lung, it may limit the heart's ability to deliver blood to the lungs, causing shortness of breath and chest pain and, in serious cases, death. Pulmonary embolism is the most preventable cause of death among hospitalized patients. Some risk factors for pulmonary embolism include obesity, smoking, cancer, pregnancy, us birth control pills or recent surgery

The signs and symptoms of pulmonary embolism are vague and may be confused with other cardio-pulmonary conditions. Some of the symptoms include shortness of breath, increased heart rate, swelling of one leg, a feeling of your heart pounding or sudden chest pain.

There are certain medications that may prevent clots from forming. These medications are called anticoagulants (blood thinners). Anticoagulants are the mainstay treatment for pulmonary embolism that work by breaking down clots before they can form. Options for anticoagulation in patients with pulmonary embolism include intravenous heparin and injectable enoxaparin, dalteparin and fondaparinux. Oral anticoagulants for pulmonary embolism include warfarin and rivaroxaban.

Patients that have been diagnosed with pulmonary embolism receive at least 6 months of anticoagulation treatment. Many patients are advised to continue anticoagulation treatment for longer, sometimes even lifelong, if their risk of recurrent pulmonary embolism is high. For some patients with large or massive pulmonary embolism, more aggressive therapy is required. These treatments include clot-dissolving medications, invasive procedures to remove the embolus with catheters or surgery and implantation of a filter device to catch free blood clots before they reach the heart. Treating risk factors for pulmonary embolism is a critical step in preventing future blood clots. Lifestyle changes such as regular exercise, a heart-healthy diet and smoking cessation are important steps in reducing risk.

Despite therapies 3-5% of patient will continue to have clots which manifest as pulmonary hypertension and is called chronic thromboembolic disease.

Interstitial lung disease (ILD)

Interstitial lung disease is a group of disorders causing progressive scarring of lung tissue and affects the interstitium impairing the ability to get enough oxygen into the bloodstream. Most cases of ILD develop gradually and have no known cause. Once lung scarring occurs, it is generally irreversible. Medications occasionally can slow the disease

never regain full function of their lungs. Researchers
...gs, many still experimental, may eventually prove
...ating this condition.

...ors can find out what's causing the fibrosis. But in
...es, they can't find a cause. They call these cases as idiopathic
pulmonary fibrosis (IPF) or usual interstitial pneumonia (UIP).

Risk factors

Because ILD has a many causes, determining the reason for an initial
injury to lung tissue can be difficult. Scarring seems to occur when an
injury to your lungs triggers an abnormal healing response. Ordinarily, the
body regenerates just the right amount of tissue for repair. However, in
ILD, there is a defect in the repair process, which produces excess scar
tissue that increasingly interferes with lung function. Some of the many
possible contributing factors include:

- Exposure to environmental pollutants, including inorganic dust
  (asbestos, silica and hard metal dusts), organic dust (bacteria and
  animal proteins) and gases and fumes
- Radiation
- The use of certain medicines, including: Nitrofurantoin and
  Sulfasalzine, Amiodarone and Bleomycin.
- Other medical conditions such as lupus, scleroderma, rheumatoid
  arthritis, dermatomyositis, polymyositis and Sjögren's syndrome
  may result in ILD.

Diagnostic Procedures

It is important to differentiate between ILD with identifiable causes and
those lung diseases without specific cause. However the distinction is not
always possible. In some situations a patient may require lung biopsy to
establish the proper type of fibrosis. Besides a detailed medical history and
physical exam, there are some recommended tests such as a chest X-ray,
high-resolution computerized tomography (HRCT) scan or pulmonary
function tests (PFTs).

Treatments

Interstitial lung disease with identifiable causes can sometimes be treated and resolved, however, in the setting of IPF the outcome is less promising. The goals of therapy in IPF are to prevent further lung scarring, alleviate symptoms and maintain the patient's ability to remain active and to improve the quality of life. Treatment can not reverse scarring that has already occurred therefore early diagnosis and management of IPF is crucial.

The management of IPF is still evolving. Though no standardized regimen for treatment exists a combination of some of the following medications are used: corticosteroids, mycophenolate mofetil, N-acetylcysteine, azathioprine, cyclophosphamide and other chemotherapeutics. Clinical trials continue to be the biggest hope for IPF patients and these medications are anti-inflammatory and anti-angiogenic (anti-blood vessel forming)

Pirfenidone

Pirfenidone is a drug that has been approved in Europe and is being evaluated here in the United States. Pirfenidone reduces fibroblast (cells responsible for causing fibrosis) proliferation and the production of fibrogenic mediators such as TGF-β in the lung. Pirfenidone has also been shown to reduce production of inflammatory mediators in the lung thus is also considered a anti-inflammatory agent.

Nintedanib

Nintedanib is a drug that inhibits the process of blood vessel formation (angiogenesis) in fibrotic centers. Angiogenesis inhibitors stop the formation and reshaping of blood vessels in and around fibrosis centers, which reduces the blood supply, starving fribrotic cells of oxygen and nutrients leading to cell death and prevention of the spread of fibrosis. Unlike conventional chemotherapy which has a direct cell killing effect on cancer cells, angiogenesis inhibitors starve fibrotic cells of oxygen and nutrients which results in cell death.

Despite these advances in therapy and new drugs on the horizon some patients may require oxygen therapy and pulmonary rehabilitation. In advanced lung fibrosis, lung transplantation may be required.

Pulmonary Arterial Hypertension

Pulmonary arterial hypertension (PAH) is a progressive disease, which can be life-threatening. The disease is defined by sustained elevations in pulmonary artery blood pressure. This leads to restricted flow in the vessels in the lungs, which makes the right side of the heart work harder. Eventually, the right side of the heart becomes overworked and enlarged.

Advanced pulmonary hypertension patients will have symptoms of shortness of breath, which is first noticed during exercise. As the disease progresses, shortness of breath may occur even at rest. Other symptoms include fatigue, cough, dizziness, chest pain ankle swelling and fainting.

Pulmonary Hypertension Nomenclature and Classification

Pulmonary hypertension may occur in many situations and be conveniently categorized into 5 groups (Table 2)

Diagnostic Testing in PAH

In addition to a detailed medical history and examination your physician may perform some of the following recommend tests:

Imaging
- Chest X Ray (CXR)
- Ventilation perfusion scanning
- Contrast computer tomography (CT Angiography) of the pulmonary arteries

Pulmonary
- Arterial blood gases
- Pulmonary function testing
- Nocturnal oxygen saturation monitoring
- Cardio-pulmonary exercise test and six-minute walk test

Cardiology
- Electrocardiogram (ECG)
- Echocardiography (screening test)
- Cardiac catheterization (gold standard for diagnosis)

Blood

- Routine hematology and biochemistry
- Thrombophilia screen
- Autoimmune screen, HIV testing

Treatments Available for Pulmonary Arterial Hypertension

In the early course of the disease, patients may be treated with oral medications, such as calcium channel blockers, endothelin receptor blockers or phosphodiesterase inhibitors. Some patients may require additional inhaled prostacyclin therapies in combination with their oral medications. Many patients may also require home oxygen therapy, diuretics (water pills) and oral anticoagulation therapy. As the disease progresses, patients may need to be placed on a life-long intravenous therapy or subcutaneous continuous infusion pump.

Treatment options for pulmonary arterial hypertension have greatly improved over the last decade. With the development of new therapies in the pipeline such as Riociguat and Mecitentan, the future for patients with pulmonary arterial hypertension is improving.

Table 2: Pulmonary Hypertension Classification–Dana Point (2008)

Group I (Pulmonary Arterial Hypertension PAH)	Idiopathic PAH (IPAH) Heritable PAH Drug and toxin-induced Associated with (APAH) • Connective tissue disease • HIV infection • Portal Hypertension • Congenital heart Disease
Group II	Systolic and Diastolic Dysfunction (Heart Failure) Valvular disease
Group III	Chronic Obstructive Pulmonary Disease (COPD) Interstitial Lung Disease (ILD) Obstructive Sleep Apnea (OSA)
Group IV	Chronic Thromboembolic Pulmonary Hypertension (CTEPH)
Group V	Miscellaneous • Hematologic disorders, splenectomy • Systemic disorders, lymphangioleimyomatosis • Metabolic disorders, thyroid disorders • Other: chronic renal failure on dialysis

Chapter 3

Diagnosing Your Disease

"Natural forces within us are the true healers of disease."

Hippocrates (460 BC – 377 BC)

In the following section, we will discuss information on different tests that your physician may order to help diagnose your heart and lung disease.

Spirometry

Spirometry is a routinely performed breathing test that assesses how well your lungs function. During this test, you will be asked to blow into a tube which is connected to a machine. This machine, or a spirometer, measures how much air your lungs can hold (forced vital capacity or FVC) and how fast you can blow air out (forced expiratory volume in one second or FEV_1). Along with a doctor's examination, spirometry can help determine how severe your COPD is. Values are expressed as percentage (%) of predicted. Predicted values are determined from your age, sex and height.

Pulmonary Function Testing (PFTs)

Pulmonary function testing is a commonly used test, ordered by the physician to evaluate the function of lungs. This testing involves the use of machinery to perform breathing tests to measure the size of lungs, the state of the airways of the lungs and the ability of the lungs to exchange oxygen and carbon dioxide.

Patients are asked to withhold long acting lung medications for 12 hours and short acting lung medications for 4 hours prior to testing. Patients are asked not to engage in vigorous physical exercise at least 4 hours prior to testing. Patients may be asked for a sample of blood to be drawn for measuring the amount of the oxygen and carbon dioxide of the blood;

done by a certified Respiratory Therapist using local anesthetic called lidocaine to numb the area over the artery in which the needle is inserted. Patients may be asked to inhale medication to open the airways in the lungs. This allows the doctors to determine how well the lungs respond to the type of medication.

6 Minute Walk Test (6MWT)

A 6MWT is a test used to find out how much you are able to exercise. The test will measure how far you can walk on a flat surface in 6 minutes. This test will allow your physician or respiratory therapist to determine your exercise capacity.

Cardio-Pulmonary Exercise Test

Another very important method for assessing prognosis in advanced lung disease is cardiopulmonary exercise testing (CPET). CPET involves measurement of oxygen consumption and carbon dioxide exhalation during exercise. Based on the results of this test and measurements of oxygen consumption your physician can better gauge how your disease is progressing and how to further manage your advanced lung disease.

Methacholine Challenge Test

Methacholine is a drug that causes narrowing of the airways. The degree of narrowing can be quantified by performing a spirometry. People with a history of hyperreactive airways such as asthmatics, will react to lower doses of drug. In addition to assessing the reversibility of a particular condition, a medication (bronchodilator) is administered to counteract the effects of the methacholine before repeating the spirometry tests. This is commonly referred to as a reversibility test and may help in distinguishing asthma from chronic obstructive pulmonary disease.

Bronchoscopy

Bronchoscopy is a common diagnostic procedure, usually done in an outpatient setting that allows your doctor to look inside your lungs and is routinely used for biopsies of shadows or changes on x-rays or CT scans. The bronchoscope is a thin, flexible tube with a tiny camera on the end and is inserted through the nose or mouth into the lungs. Bronchoscopy is a safe diagnostic procedure and carries little risk.

How to Prepare for Bronchoscopy?

Do not eat or drink for six to eight hours before the procedure (not even water). It is important that your stomach be empty to avoid aspiration (vomiting).

You may take important medications with a sip of water. Please discuss with your pulmonologist which medications you may take prior to the procedure and if you are on any blood thinners, such as: Plavix, Coumadin, Aspirin and/or Aspirin-containing products.

Bring a list of your current medications, past medical history and surgeries. To have the procedure, you will need a responsible adult to stay with you before, during and after the procedure to drive you home.

Complications are infrequent, but if they occur, they may include pneumothorax (collapsed lung), bleeding at the biopsy site and allergic reaction to medications.

Abdominal Aortic Aneurysm ultrasound

A test that measures the size of the major artery that is located in the stomach area. This test is recommended 1 times only for men aged 65-75 years who have ever smoked.

Angiogram or Arteriogram

In an angiogram or arteriogram dye is injected into the blood vessels using a catheter (small tube) and X-rays are taken. This test shows whether arteries are narrowed or blocked. A coronary angiogram checks for narrowing or blockages in the blood vessels that go to the heart. A cerebral arteriogram checks the blood vessels that go to the brain.

Angioplasty

Angioplasty also called balloon angioplasty is a procedure used to remove a blockage in a blood vessel to the heart (coronary angioplasty) or the brain. A small tube with a balloon attached is threaded into the narrowed or blocked blood vessel. Then the balloon is inflated, opening the narrowed artery. A wire tube, called a stent, may be left in place to help keep the artery open.

Ankle Brachial Index

A test called an ankle brachial index or ABI is used to diagnose peripheral artery disease (PAD). Health care providers compare the blood pressure in the ankle with that in the arm. Lower blood pressure in the lower part of the leg compared with the pressure in the arm may indicate PAD.

Cardiac catheterization

Left heart cardiac catheterization is used in conjunction with other tests. A small tube is inserted into an artery and guided into the blood vessel of the heart. It helps to locate blockages in the heart vessels and allows your cardiologist to perform on the spot angioplasty.

Right Heart Catheterization

Here in a small tube is passed in the right side of the heart to measure the pressures in the pulmonary artery. This is the gold standard test for diagnosing pulmonary artery hypertension.

Chest X Ray

A chest X-ray shows the size and shape of the heart and can also show congestion in the lungs.

Coronary Artery Bypass Graft (CABG)

During a coronary artery bypass graft, also called a bypass or CABG (pronounced "cabbage"), a blood vessel taken from the leg, wrist, or chest is attached to the coronary artery to bypass a blockage and restore blood flow to the heart. A bypass graft can also be used for blood vessels leading to the brain.

CAT (Computed Axial Tomography) Scan

A CAT scan uses special scanning techniques to provide images of the lungs. You may be given a contrast prior to the test then this study is called as CT Angiography. This test allows your physician to evaluate your pulmonary arteries to look for any clots in them.

Dual X-ray Absorptiometry (DEXA)

DEXA is a test to screen for bone health in the elderly. DEXA uses low dose radiation to measure bone density in the spine, hip and whole body. According to the World Health Organization, osteoporosis is defined as bone mineral density standard deviation score (BMD-T) < 2.5; a bone density in this low range predicts future fracture risk. In children and adolescents, the use of a BMD-T is inappropriate and a BMD-Z must be used. How well BMD-Z predicts fracture risk in younger individuals is less well established. Thus, osteoporosis is defined in children and younger adults as BMD-Z<-2 and a history of significant fractures, including long bone fractures of the upper and lower extremities and compression fractures of the spine. For those on steroid therapy it is important to have a DEXA scan on a yearly basis for those that are on steroid therapy such as prednisone.

Echocardiogram

An echocardiogram uses high-frequency sound waves (ultrasound) to produce images of the heart and blood vessels. Results indicate whether the heart is pumping blood correctly. It also allows us to estimate the pressure in the pulmonary arteries. This is good screening test when your health care provider wants to rule out pulmonary artery hypertension. A stress echocardiogram uses either exercise or medication and ultrasound to provide images of the heart and blood vessels under stress.

Electrocardiogram (EKG, ECG)

An electrocardiogram, also called an ECG or EKG, provides information on heart rate and rhythm and shows whether there has been any damage or injury to the heart muscle.

Exercise Perfusion Test (Nuclear Cardiac Stress Test)

An exercise perfusion test uses small amounts of radioactive material to produce images of blood flow to the heart as you exercise.

Exercise Stress Test

Exercise stress tests are used to find heart disease that is evident only during physical activity. It can also be used to help a patient choose the most appropriate physical activity program. Also called a treadmill test, a stress test uses an ECG to measure how the heart performs during activity, such as walking on a moving treadmill. A medication stress test uses medication instead of exercise to increase the heart rate.

Holter Monitoring

A Holter monitor is a small, portable machine that records the heart's electrical activity. The person wearing the monitor keeps track of symptoms and activities for the evaluation period. Readings on the machine are compared with the symptoms.

Magnetic Resonance Imaging (MRI)

MRI uses special scanning techniques to provide images of body tissues. MRA (magnetic resonance angiography) uses MRI to examine blood vessels.

Nuclear Ventriculography

Nuclear ventriculography also called radionuclide ventriculography uses small amounts of radioactive material to check heart function either while the body is at rest or during exercise. This test can also be used to check the blood vessels that go to the brain.

Ventilation Perfusion Scan

In this test, small amounts of radioactive material are injected in to the veins to evaluate the flow of blood through the lungs. This test is generally used to help diagnose presence of clots in the lungs, which are known as pulmonary embolism.

Positron Emission Tomography (PET)

A PET scan uses special scanning techniques to provide images of body tissues. It helps to identify any tissue in the body that may be cancerous.

Chapter 4

Pulmonary Medications

"The best doctor gives the least medicines."

Benjamin Franklin (1706-1790)

There are many different types of prescribed medications that may help you breathe easier. Your doctor may have already prescribed some of these for you. This section is designed to help you understand why you're taking a particular medication, how the various medications work and if there are any possible side effects. You should always tell your doctor if you are taking any other medications (which should only be used under the direction of your physician). This is particularly true of narcotics, sleeping pills, or tranquilizers.

How to take medications safely

Since many patients are on multiple medications at times, there may be interactions amongst these medications. This may result in unwanted reactions. Such interactions may result from:

- Two medications such as aspirin and blood thinners
- Drugs and food such as statins and grapefruit
- Drug supplements, such as gingko biloba and blood thinners
- Drugs and other diseases, such as aspirin and peptic ulcer disease
- Food and beverages may interact poorly with medicines

Some common things to watch for

Alcohol: Avoid alcohol, it can increase or decrease the effect of many drugs.

Grapefruit juice: This juice should not be taken with certain blood pressure lowering medications. This juice can cause higher levels of those medications in your body, making it more likely that you will have side effects from these medications.

Licorice: This also would reduce the effects of blood pressure medications, as well as diuretics. Licorice may increase the level of Digoxin, a common medication used to treat congestive heart failure.

Chocolate: It is contraindicated with certain types of anti depressants called MAO inhibitors. Caffeine in chocolate can interact with stimulant medications like Ritalin (methylphenidate), increasing their effect or by decreasing the effect of sedative hypnotics such as Ambien (Zolpidem)

Preventing Medication Errors

Know your medication: Keep a list of all your medications, how much you take and when you take. Include over the counter medicines, vitamins, supplements and herbs. Take this list to all your doctor visits. Keep this list current all the times. Never take medications prescribed for others. Ask your healthcare provider if you do not know the answer to these questions. Please ask your doctor or pharmacist the following:

- Why am I taking this medication?
- What are the common problems to watch for?
- What should I do if they occur?
- When should I stop this medicine?
- Can I take this medication with the other medicines on my list?

Expectorants and Mucolytics (Decongestants)

These drugs are designed to increase removal of respiratory tract fluids and help liquefy mucus that is sticky or thick. They're available in liquids, elixirs, drops, liquid capsules and liquid for inhalation only. Some examples are water, Guaifenesin, Iodide Humibid, Acetylcysteine (Mucomyst®)

Drinking fluids is the best way to liquefy mucus. Expectorants should not be combined with antihistamines such as Benadryl® or cough suppressants like codeine or dextromethorphan. Mucomyst should be used with a bronchodilator. Once opened, it is good for 96 hours and should be refrigerated. Rinse mouth after use to eliminate aftertaste.

Aspirin

Individuals with asthma or asthma symptoms might find that aspirin causes excessive shortness of breath and wheezing. If this occurs, discuss a substitute with your physician. There are a variety of aspirin substitutes on the market today.

Antibiotics

Antibiotics help fight existing bacterial infections and help prevent future severe infections. There are hundreds of different types and your physician will make the decision on which one is the best for your specific situation. Antibiotics are available in tablets, capsules, liquids and injections in the vein (intravenous-IV). Examples: Ampicillin, Erythromycin, Penicillin, Tetracycline, Bactrim®, Zithromax®, Levaquin®, Biaxin®, Avelox®, Amoxicillin. (See Appendix 1)

Possible side effects of antibiotics may be upset stomach or allergic reactions; nausea, vomiting or diarrhea. There may be other side effects as specified by your doctor.

Bronchodilators

Bronchodilators relax muscles around the airways to keep them open, making it easier to breathe. They're available in tablets, elixirs, inhalants, suppositories and injections. Examples: Albuterol (Proventil®/Ventolin®), Serevent®, Aminophylline, Ephedrine, Epinephrine, Maxair® Isoproterenol (Isuprel; Isuprel Mistometer) Metaproterenol (Alupent®; Metaprel®) Terbutaline (Brethine; Bricanyl), Theophylline, Brovana® (Arformoterol) and Xopenex® (Levosalbutamol). Some of these medications may be available in inhaler form however some may be available in nebulizer form as well. Possible side effects are increased heart rate; anxiety; nervousness; shakiness; headaches; upset stomach; heartburn; loss of appetite; sleeplessness and sweating. (See Appendix 2)

Cromolyn Sodium

Cromolyn prevents bronchial asthma attacks and inhibits allergic/asthmatic reactions. The side effects include possible occasional coughing and wheezing; skin rash, itching; and nausea. Cromolyn is available in powder or liquid for inhalation only. To reduce the possibility of coughing and wheezing, a bronchodilator should be used before inhaling cromolyn sodium. It is important to note that cromolyn can help prevent an asthma attack but it will not help in an acute attack of asthma.

Steroids

Steroids decrease airway swelling and inflammation. They help decrease wheezing by allowing the airways to remain relaxed and open. They're available in tablets, inhalers and intravenous form. Oral steroids are prednisone and methylpednisolone (Medrol®). Inhaled steroids are QVar® (beclomethasone), Aerobid® (Flunisolide), Azmacort® (Triamcinolone), Flovent® (Fluticasone) and Pulmicort® (Budesonide)

Possible side effects of oral steroids are weight gain and puffiness due to fluid retention; stomach ache; fragile bones; skin bruises easily; lowers your resistance to infections. Inhalers may cause dry mouth, hoarseness and oral-dental fungal infections. It is important to remember not to discontinue or change the dosage of steroids on your own. Changes should only be made by your physician and usually will involve a gradual taper. Take oral steroid medications with food, milk, or antacids to ease possible stomach problems. After using inhalers, rinse your mouth to avoid any irritation and infection.

Combination of Steroids and Bronchodilators

There are options that combine Steroids and Bronchodilators into one inhaler or nebulizer. This allows for an anti-inflammatory effect as well as a treatment to open the airways in one medication. Some examples are Advair® (fluticasone/salmeterol), Symbicort® (budesonide/formoterol) and DuoNeb® (ipratropium bromide/salbutamol)

Diuretics (water pills)

Since diuretics help rid the body of excess fluids, they may cause mucus membranes to dry out. Thick, sticky mucus is harder to cough up and creates an environment for bacterial growth. If you are taking water pills for another condition, you should contact your physician. It is possible your doctor will supplement your potassium while you are on water pills.

Anticoagulants (blood thinners) for Venous Thromboembolism

If someone is ever diagnosed with a clot in their lungs called a pulmonary embolism they will be initiated on anticoagulant therapy. Most commonly patients are started with warfarin (Coumadin®). For people who are unable to tolerate warfarin or unable to comply with frequent laboratory testing there are alternatives.

An alternative to warfarin is the oral anticoagulant rivaroxaban (Xarelto®). It is the first available orally active direct factor Xa (clotting factor) inhibitor. It is well absorbed from the gut and the effect lasts 8–12 hours. The one downside of rivaroxaban is that there is no specific way to reverse the anticoagulant effect of rivaroxaban in the event of a major bleeding event, unlike warfarin.

Dabigatran (Pradaxa®) for Arterial Thromboembolism

Another anti-coagulant, used for cardiac manifestations such as atrial fibrillation and arterial clots is dabigatran (Pradaxa®). It is an oral anticoagulant from the class of the direct thrombin inhibitors. One of the benefits is that it does not require frequent blood tests while offering similar results in terms of efficacy. One downside of dabigatran is that there is no specific way to reverse the anticoagulant effect of in the event of a major bleeding event.

Antivirals to Prevent and Treat Flu

While the Centers for Disease Control and Prevention (CDC) recommends flu vaccination as the first and most important step in preventing the flu, antiviral drugs are a second line of defense. Two medications Oseltamivir (Tamiflu®) and Zanamvir (Relenza®) are recommended to treat and prevent flu infection. The medications are different from antibiotics and are not sold over the counter; you can only get them if you have a prescription from your doctor. While most people with flu have mild illness that resolve over time some patients may benefit from antivirals. A physician's clinical judgment is most important in deciding if antiviral drugs are needed to treat flu infection. The medications are most effective if started within 2 days of flu symptoms. Antivirals can make one feel better and shorten the duration of symptoms. They can also prevent serious complications, such as pneumonia. These medications are taken for 5 days but hospitalized patients may need the medicine for longer duration.

Vaccinations

Vaccines play an important role in health maintenance of patients with advanced lung disease. (See Appendix 3)

Flu Vaccine - A seasonal vaccine is distributed routinely every year. Generally everyone 6 month or older should get vaccinated against the flu. Most people who get flu do not need any therapy and generally recover within two weeks. Some people are more likely to get complications like pneumonia, bronchitis, sinus infection and ear infections. The flu can also make chronic health problems like asthma, heart failure and diabetes worse. Listed below is the group of people more likely to get flu related complications if they get sick from influenza.

Persons at increased risk for flu-related complications include:

- Persons >65 years of age
- Residents of chronic care facilities housing persons of any age with chronic medical conditions
- Persons with chronic cardiopulmonary disease, including children with asthma, COPD
- Persons requiring regular medical care for chronic diseases, including diabetes mellitus, kidney or liver dysfunction, or blood disorders (Sickle cell disease)
- Persons with weakened immune system (e.g. HIV)
- People who are morbidly obese (Body Mass Index >40)
- Health care workers (physicians, nurses) and other people who live or care for high risk people to keep from spreading flu to high risk people

Pneumococcal Vaccine

Pneumonia caused by bacteria *Streptococcus pneumoniae* (pneumococcus) is particularly notorious for causing significant morbidity and mortality. Pneumococcal vaccine is effective at preventing severe disease, hospitalization and death. However, it is not guaranteed to prevent symptomatic infection in everyone. Adults, 65 years of age or older and children younger than 5 years of age are more prone to pneumonia infection. People up to 64 years of age who have underlying medical conditions such as diabetes, HIV/AIDS and people 19 through 64 who smoke or have asthma are also at increased risk for getting pneumonia.

Pneumovax® is 23-valent polysaccharide vaccine (PPVSV) that is currently recommended for use in all adults who are older than 65 years of age and for persons who are 2 years and older and at high risk for disease (e.g., sickle cell disease, HIV infection, or other immuno-compromising conditions like cardiovascular diseases, chronic pulmonary diseases, diabetes mellitus, alcoholism, cirrhosis). It is also recommended for use in adults 19 through 64 years old who smoke or who have asthma.

Varicella Zoster Virus Vaccine

Herpes zoster which is commonly known as shingles is a viral disease characterized by a painful skin rash with blisters in a limited area on one side of the body often in a linear fashion. The initial infection with varicella zoster virus (VZV) causes the acute, short-lived illness chickenpox which generally occurs in children and young adults. The VZV vaccine is recommended by the Centers for Disease Control for any individual over the age of 60.

Tetanus Toxoid Vaccine

Tetanus is a medical condition characterized by prolonged contraction of skeletal muscle. The primary symptoms are caused by tetanospasmin, a neurotoxin produced by the bacteria *Clostridium tetani.* Tetanus infection generally occurs through contamination through an open wound that involves a cut or deep puncture wound. As the infection progresses, muscle spasms develop in the jaw and elsewhere in the body. Most individuals have been vaccinated at one point in their lives but it is recommended that you receive a tetanus booster every 10 years.

Chapter 5

<u>Oxygen Therapy</u>

"Water, air and cleanness are the chief articles in my pharmacy."

Napoleon I (1769-1821)

Oxygen is a basic need for all humans. The air we breathe contains about 21% oxygen. This amount is enough for people with healthy lungs and many with lung disease. However, some people with lung disease are unable to gather enough oxygen through normal breathing, so they require extra oxygen to maintain normal body function. Oxygen therapy in this set of patients improves survival and quality of life. Patients with advanced lung disease can have low levels of oxygen in their bodies and some need to use supplemental oxygen to bring their oxygen levels up to a healthier level.

How do I know if I need oxygen?

A healthcare provider will figure out if you need oxygen therapy by initially testing your oxygen level (O_2 sat) with a small device called a pulse oximeter that can be clipped painlessly on your finger or earlobe over a period of time, even during sleep or exercise. Another test to gauge the level of oxygen in your blood is called arterial blood gas (ABG) and involves taking a blood sample to determine the levels of oxygen and carbon dioxide. Patients who have a room air oxygen saturation of less than 88% or 59mmHg on room air in the presence of advanced lung disease are considered for oxygen therapy.

How much oxygen should I take?

Oxygen is a medical treatment that requires a prescription by a healthcare provider. Once the amount of oxygen needed is decided, the provider will prescribe an oxygen setting or flow rate depending on the severity of your condition. Depending on your daily activities the flow rate of your oxygen will adjust accordingly. During any physical activity, people use more energy and therefore need more oxygen. To find out how much oxygen is needed during activity, the provider will have you do an exercise stress test or a walk test while measuring your oxygen saturation. Too little or too much oxygen may be detrimental to your health so you should follow regularly with your health care provider.

Oxygen Supply Methods

In an outpatient or home setting the oxygen is supplied by one of three sources. One is compressed oxygen cylinders which may provide an oxygen flow rate of up to 15L/min. Patients requiring greater than 4L/min flow will require a humidifier to prevent the nasal mucosa from drying out. The second type of supply method is liquid oxygen systems as one cubic foot of liquid oxygen is equivalent to 860 cubic feet of gas, they can stores large amount of oxygen in small spaces. Hence this is useful for high volume users, though cost may be an issue. The other supply method is oxygen concentrator, which is an electrically powered device that takes ambient air and physically separated the oxygen from the nitrogen. This is the most cost efficient supply method at home for those who need continuous low flow oxygen. The oxygen is delivered by all three devices via a nasal cannula.

Will I always need to use oxygen?

Majority of patients who require oxygen supplementation to treat their lung disease will need to continue their oxygen therapy. Some patients may need to use extra oxygen during a disease flare-up or infection, but may be able to reduce or stop its use if their condition improves. You should never reduce or stop oxygen therapy on your own. Talk with your healthcare provider if you think a change in your oxygen therapy is needed.

If you have been prescribed oxygen, be sure to use it while exercising. If you become short of breath during exercise, it means your body needs more oxygen. To restore your normal levels of oxygen quickly, do your pursed lip breathing exercises, concentrating on exhaling, while you rest.

Chapter 6

Pulmonary Hypertension Medications

"A mortal lives not through that breath that flows in and that flows out. The source of his life is another and this causes the breath to flow."

Paracelsus (1493-1541)

In the early course of pulmonary hypertension, patients may be treated with oral medications, known as calcium channel blockers, which can lower the pulmonary artery pressure. However, newer medications, specifically developed for the treatment of pulmonary hypertension may also be prescribed. Often, patients may require diuretics and oral anticoagulation therapy. Some may even require home oxygen therapy.

Phosphodiesterase Type 5 (PDE-5) Inhibitors

Phosphodiesterase type-5 inhibitors are drugs used to block the degradative action of the enzyme phosphodiesterase type 5 on cyclic GMP in the smooth muscle cells lining the pulmonary arteries. PDE-5 inhibitors are used for the treatment of pulmonary hypertension as given below.

Revatio® (Sildenafil)

Revatio® is a PDE-5 inhibitor that contains sildenafil citrate (also known as Viagra). Revatio® helps dilate the pulmonary arteries leading to a decrease in the pulmonary artery pressure. In studies, Revatio® helped people walk increased distances. Usual dose is one table, three times a day.

As with all PDE-5 inhibitors you should not take nitrates, certain anti-virals (such as ritonavir) or anti-fungals (such as ketoconazole and itraconazole). Some possible side effects are nosebleeds, upset stomach, headache, flushing, trouble sleeping. In rare cases, a sudden decrease or loss of sight has been reported during use of this drug. Therefore, routine eye exams are essential.

Adcirca® (Tadalafil)

Adcirca® is also a PDE-5 inhibitor that only has to be taken once a day. It is used to improve exercise tolerance. It treats PAH by widening blood vessels in the lungs. As a result, blood vessels can better carry oxygen-rich blood to the rest of the body. The most common side effect of Adcirca is headache. Other common adverse events include myalgia, nasopharyngitis, flushing, respiratory tract infection, extremity pain, nausea, back pain, dyspepsia and nasal congestion.

Endothelin Receptor Antagonists (ERAs)

Endothelin (ET) system especially ET_1 and the ET_A and ET_B receptors have been implicated in the pathogenesis of PAH. Endothelin receptor antagonists are drugs that block endothelin receptors that are present in the lining of the pulmonary vasculature.

Tracleer® (Bosentan)

Tracleer® is an endothelin receptor blocker that blocks the ET_A and ET_B receptors. Endothelin in a large amount contributes to the tightening of blood vessels. Tracleer® helps to block the harmful effects of endothelin, to improve blood flow and decrease pulmonary artery pressure. Tracleer® has been shown to improve symptoms and improve ability to perform daily activities.

While on Tracleer® should not be taken with cyclosporine A or glyburide. These medications can cause excessive levels of Tracleer® to stay in your blood and increase your chance of liver damage.

Possible side effects are headaches, flushing or hot flashes, leg/ankle swelling, low blood pressure, inflammation of the throat and nasal passages. As Tracleer® may cause liver damage; therefore monthly liver monitoring is necessary. Tracleer® can cause birth defects; therefore patients on Tracleer® cannot be or become pregnant. Women starting therapy will require a serum pregnancy test initially and monthly (if applicable). They are also advised to utilize a double barrier method of contraception.

Letairis® (Ambrisentan)

Letairis® is an endothelin receptor antagonist but is a more selective blocker of the ET_A receptor. It can help to improve blood flow and decrease pulmonary artery pressure. Letairis® can improve your ability to exercise it helps slow down the worsening of your physical condition and symptoms. If you are on cyclosporine or similar medications, it may slow down how quickly your body processes Ambrisentan.

Possible side effects are lowering of red blood cell count, swelling of legs and ankles (edema), stuffy nose (nasal congestion), or getting red in the face (flushing), feeling your heart beat (palpitations) and visual disturbances.

Letairis® can cause birth defects; therefore patients on Letairis® cannot be or become pregnant. Women starting therapy will require a serum pregnancy test initially and monthly (if applicable).

Opsumit® (Macitentan)

Macitentan is an ERA that has been recently approved for the treatment of pulmonary arterial hypertension. Like medications mentioned before Macitentan is an endothelin receptor blocker that works on two kinds of chemical receptors that control the dilation of the blood vessels in your lungs. It has been shown to be more effective than Bosentan while causing less irritation to the liver. Women starting therapy will require a serum pregnancy test initially and monthly (if applicable).

Prostacyclin Analogues

Prostacyclin is an endogenous substance that is produced by vascular endothelial cells and induces vasodilatation. A malfunction of prostacyclin metabolic pathways has been shown in patients with PAH and this represents the rationale for the exogenous therapeutic administration of prostacyclin analogues given below.

Remodulin® (Intravenous Treprostinil)

Remodulin® is a prostacyclin vasodilator indicated for the treatment of PAH to diminish symptoms associated with exercise. Remodulin® can be delivered by a small, discrete pump through either continuous subcutaneous (SC) infusion or continuous intravenous (IV) infusion. It has a four-hour half-life and is stable at temperatures up to 104° F, so there's no need for ice packs. Possible side effects are: catheter infections, flushing, jaw pain and stomach discomfort.

Tyvaso® (Inhaled Treprostinil)

Tyvaso® is a synthetic form of prostacyclinused to treat pulmonary arterial hypertension. The drug is delivered by inhalation and should only be used with the Tyvaso inhalation system.If you are taking Gemfibrozil or Rifampicin, then the doses of Tyvaso® may need to be adjusted. The most common side effects of Tyvaso are coughing, headache, throat irritation, pain, nausea, reddening of the face and neck (flushing) and fainting or loss of consciousness.

Orenitram® (Oral Treprostinil)

Orenitram® is an approved oral form of treprostinil and has been approved as a first line therapy for patients exhibiting functional class II or III symptoms. It has also been planned to be used as an adjuvant therapy in patients where monotherapy with other first line oral medications are not therapeutic. Side effects and adverse events are similar to inhaled and intravenous treprostinil.

Flolan® (Epoprostenol)

Flolan® or epoprostenol is a synthetic form of a naturally occurring molecule in the human body called prostaglandin which helps the body open blood vessels. This synthetic substance is called prostacyclin. Flolan® is administered intravenously directly into the bloodstream through a surgically implanted catheter by a portable, battery-operated pump. Since the drug lasts only 3-5 minutes it must constantly be infused: it is slowly and continuously pumped into the body through the permanent catheter placed in a vein in the neck or chest. The pump is filled daily with the mixed Flolan® solution. It is important to remember that this medication cannot be abruptly stopped. Common side effects are flushing, headache, jaw pain, stomach discomfort and joint pain.

Veletri® (Epoprostenol)

Veletri® is the brand name of a drug whose key ingredient is epoprostenol, which is a prostacyclin. Veletri® unlike Flolan® does not require ice packs and you don't need special mixing liquids (diluents) to prepare your medicine

Ventavis® (Inhaled Iloprost)

Iloprost is a synthetic analogue of prostacyclin and it works by dilating the blood vessels. It is delivered via inhalation, with a 1-Neb device, a breath-actuated pulmonary drug delivery device. Some possible side effects include dizziness, lightheadedness, fainting, flushing, increased cough, low blood pressure, headaches and nausea.

Adempas® (Riociguat)

Riociguat is a recently approved medication by the Food and Drug Administration for treatment of chronic thromboembolic pulmonary hypertension (CTEPH) and PAH. This medication is a stimulator of soluble guanylate cyclase (sGC) which is a receptor for the vasodilator, nitric oxide. It has been shown to increase exercise tolerance and functional capacity. Side effects include upset stomach and sudden drop in blood pressure

Chapter 7

Pulmonary Rehabilitation

"Walking is man's best medicine."

Hippocrates (460 BC – 377 BC)

Starting a pulmonary rehabilitation program is more than just physical therapy. There are classes which address subjects such as medication administration, stress management and smoking cessation. Pulmonary rehab can help anyone to manage their symptoms and slow the progression of lung disease. While results vary from person to person, the ultimate goal is to increase your independence, decrease your hospitalizations and improve your quality of life.

Pulmonary Rehabilitation Means

- Fewer hospitalizations
- Improved activities of daily living
- Nutritional awareness
- Educational awareness
- Shortness of breath reduction

Emotional and Physical Rewards of Exercising

- Improves blood flow circulation and improves oxygen delivery to the body
- Decreases stress hormones
- These changes help ward off depression

What should I expect in pulmonary rehabilitation?

Structure of pulmonary rehabilitation programs can vary from center to center. The majority of programs are held as group classes, while others are done individually. Most programs encourage family and friends to attend with you. Keep in mind that you should always consult a doctor before attempting a new or modified exercise program, especially if you are not currently active.

Before you begin, a pulmonary rehabilitation team member will meet with you to talk about your chronic lung disease and its physical and emotional effect on you. You may have to take a short quiz about lung diseases and may be asked to set goals for your progress. For your first class, wear comfortable clothing and walking shoes. Make sure to bring your fast-acting inhaler, supplemental oxygen equipment and other prescribed medications.

Prior to initiation of pulmonary rehabilitation a staff member will measure the distance you are able to walk in six minutes (6 minute walk test) while a device called a pulse oximeter determines the oxygen saturation in your blood through a sensor on your finger or forehead. The test results will help the rehabilitation team assess your functional exercise capacity and develop an exercise program tailored to your abilities.

Exercise Training

As your weeks of pulmonary rehabilitation progress, you will practice a regimen of stretching, aerobic activities like walking and strength exercises using free weights and resistance bands. A typical exercise program emphasizes endurance training for 30 to 40 minutes repeated at least three times weekly, but preferably five to seven times a week.

It is important to exercise at home as well. This "homework" includes walking, stretching, weight lifting, bicycling, swimming, or performing other activities recommended by your rehabilitation team. Keep up this routine even after completing rehabilitation to ensure its long-term effectiveness. Patients who discontinue exercise following rehabilitation typically return to their previous state of health within 12 to 18 months.

The rehabilitation team will also show you how to conserve energy and pace yourself during exercise and daily activities. They will demonstrate strategies to help reduce your shortness of breath.

Keep up to date on your vaccinations.

While at the physician's office take an active approach and ensure that all of your vaccinations are up to date as well as your medication refills. It is important for anyone with advanced lung disease to stay up to date on their vaccinations to prevent further complications of their existing condition. (See Appendix 3).

Breathing Exercises

Pursed Lip Breathing & Diaphragmatic Breathing

Many people with chronic lung disease find themselves getting less exercise. They think that being breathless and tired must mean the activity is harming their lungs and heart and that it is better to be resting. This is not true. If you don't exercise, your muscles weaken and you become less able to do the things you want to do. When you exercise any muscles regularly, they are able to do more work on less oxygen. It is important to stay as active as you can. By doing these breathing exercises, you will be able to do more before having to stop because you are short of breath. The goals of breathing exercises are to:

- Improve abdominal breathing and the function of the diaphragm.
- Control respiratory rate and decrease the work of breathing.
- Assist in relaxation and thereby alleviate dyspnea.
- Increase the strength, coordination and efficiency of breathing patterns.
- Prevent or reverse atelectasis (lung collapse).
- Mobilize and maintain mobility of the chest wall.

Pursed-Lip Breathing

Pursed-lip breathing is effective in reducing the respiratory rate and relieving dyspnea. It has been suggested that this method of breathing may improve ventilation and oxygenation.

- Relax your neck and shoulder muscles.
- Inhale slowly through your nose for at least 2 counts.
- Pucker your lips as if to blowout a candle.
- Exhale slowly and gently through your pursed lips for at least twice as long as you inhaled.

Therapeutic objectives

- Alleviate difficulty in breathing and decrease respiratory rate
- Increase tolerance to exercise and strengthen muscles

Physiological objectives

- Increase alveolar ventilation
- Increase oxygenation
- Reduce work of breathing
- Decrease carbon dioxide pressure

Potential outcomes

- Strengthen core muscles
- Increased arterial oxygen pressure
- Decreased carbon dioxide pressure
- Increased exercise tolerance

COPD patients frequently use pursed-lip breathing spontaneously. Two methods of pursed-lip breathing have been reported. The preferred method advocates passive expiration and the other suggests abdominal muscle contraction through expiration. In the latter patients must be taught not to exhale forcefully, since this method increases bronchiolar collapse. You can practice breathing this way anytime, anywhere. If you're watching TV, practice during the commercials. Try to practice several times a day. Over time, pursed-lip breathing will feel natural.

- Use pursed-lip breathing to prevent shortness of breath when you do things such as exercising, climbing stairs and bending or lifting.
- Breathe out during the difficult part of any activity, such as when you bend, lift, or reach.
- Always breathe out for longer than you breathe in. This allows your lungs to empty as much as possible.
- Never hold your breath when doing pursed-lip breathing.

Diaphragmatic Breathing

The diaphragm is the most efficient muscle of breathing. It is a large, dome-shaped muscle located at the base of the lungs. Your abdominal muscles help move the diaphragm and give you more power to empty your lungs. COPD may prevent the diaphragm from working effectively. When you have pulmonary disease, air often becomes trapped in the lungs, pushing down on the diaphragm. The neck and chest muscles then have an increased share of the work of breathing. This can leave the diaphragm weakened and flattened, causing it to work less efficiently. Diaphragmatic breathing is intended to help you use the diaphragm correctly while breathing to:

- Strengthen the diaphragm muscle
- Decrease the work of breathing by slowing your breathing rate
- Decrease oxygen demand
- Use less effort and energy to breathe

Diaphragmatic Breathing Technique

- If you have a prescribed inhaled bronchodilator, take this medication before starting diaphragmatic breathing exercise.
- Lie flat with your head tilted up, or sit comfortably, with your knees bent and your shoulders, head and neck relaxed.
- Place one hand on your stomach just at the base or end of your breastbone. This hand will tell you when your diaphragm presses down against your abdomen, pushing your stomach out.
- Place your other hand on your upper chest. Use this hand to tell you how much movement is occurring in your chest muscles.
- Inhale slowly through your nose and allow your stomach to expand outward. Feel the pressure in your stomach; try to keep the upper chest from moving.
- Exhale slowly, remembering to use purse-lip breathing.
- Try to use only your diaphragm, pulling your abdomen in as much as you can.
- Include rest periods.
- Repeat this exercise until you feel comfortable using diaphragmatic and purse-lip breathing together, lying down and

then practice exercises sitting. Afterward, try exercises in standing and then leaning forward, positions.

Physical Exercises

Stretching and Strengthening Exercises

Stretching Flexibility Program - Unless otherwise noted, each stretch should be performed 3 times a week and held for 30 seconds. Refrain from bouncing or jerky movements. A rest period of 5 seconds is sufficient between each repetition. While performing these stretches you may experience some minor discomfort, or even a mild "burn", within the muscle. No joint pain should be experienced. If any pain is felt in the joint, discontinue the exercise and consult your therapist.

Flexibility exercises - These exercises should be performed 5 times per week prior to your lower extremity exercises (treadmill, stationary-bike, or free walking).

Lower Body Exercise Endurance Program - Stretching exercises should be performed prior to your lower body work out and a cool-down immediately following exercise for approximately 3 minutes. Begin exercising for 10 minutes daily then increase to 20 minutes. After you perform 30 minutes of continuous exercise, increase the intensity. Your goal is to complete 30 minutes of continuous exercise. If you are performing free walking, remember to walk with your arms hanging loosely, your chest and shoulders relaxed. Lower body exercises should be performed 5 times a week.

Upper Body and Strength Training Program - Arm raises seated in a chair should be performed initially for 10 minutes without weights. When you are able to complete 10 minutes of continuous exercise, add ½-1.0 lb weights to your routine. Therabands (elastic bands) or free weights can be used to strengthen your body. You should perform 5-6 different exercises for both the upper and lower body. Each exercise should be performed initially only 10 times per set. Gradually increase to 20-30 times per set and then increase intensity. All strengthening exercises should be done in a slow, controlled manner. Avoid any explosive or sharp movements, as this can strain your muscles and your breathing. Upper body and strength training should be performed 3 times a week.

Below is a sample physical exercise regimen which can help. Keep in mind that your exercise plan should be reviewed by your physician to ensure that you are not putting yourself at any risk of injury. Durations and weight limits should be decided after a consultation with a physical therapist, respiratory therapist and your physician.

Do NOT hold your breath during these exercises. Inhale through your nose and exhale through pursed lips as you exert force.

Stretching Exercises

The following exercises are designed to gradually increase the strength of various muscle groups. Strengthening of your muscle will help with your overall health but most importantly it will help streamline your lung function. All exercises should be initially performed under supervision. Weightlifting exercises should be performed using a comfortable amount of weight; remember not to exert yourself. They may be repeated in sets of 3 or whatever you feel comfortable doing.

Cervical Spine and Neck

Flexibility of Neck

Exercise 1

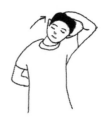

- Place hand on same side shoulder blade
- With other hand gently stretch head down and away
- Hold for 3 seconds

Exercise 2

- Gently grasp side of head while reaching behind back with other hand
- Tilt head away until a gentle stretch is felt
- Hold for 3 seconds

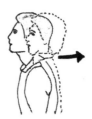

Flexibility: Neck Retraction

- Pull head straight back keeping jaw and eyes level
- Hold for 3 seconds

Cervical Spine - Phase I: Shoulder Shrugs

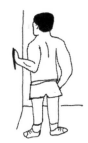

- Shrug shoulders up and down, forward and backward
- Hold for one second

Flexibility: Corner Stretch

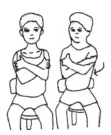

- Standing in corner with hands at shoulder level and feet a comfortable distance from the corner, lean forward until a comfortable stretch is felt across chest
- Hold for 2 seconds

Phase II: Resistive Shoulder Shrugs

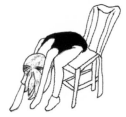

- With surgical tubing/dumbbells, shrug shoulders up and down, forward and backward

Back - Lumbar Rotation in Sitting

- Gently rotate trunk side to side in a small, pain-free motion

Back - Seated Low Back Stretch

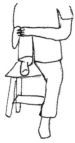

- Sit in chair with knees spread apart. Bend forward to floor
- A comfortable stretch should be felt in lower back

Hip and Knee - Standing Hamstring Stretch

* Pull knee toward chest until easy stretch is felt

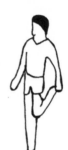

Calf Stretch

* Straighten leg out in front of you
* Bring your toes back toward your knee as you push your heel forward

Hip and Knee - Gastrocnemius Stretch

* Keeping back leg straight, with heel on floor and turned slightly outward, lean into wall until a stretch is felt in calf

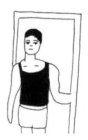

Hip and Knee - Soleus Stretch

* Keeping back leg slightly bent, with heel on floor and turned slightly outward, lean into wall until a stretch is felt in calf

Quadriceps Stretch

* Pull heel toward buttock until a stretch is felt in front of thigh

Shoulder - Range of Motion Exercises (Self-stretching activities)

External Rotation (alternate)

* Keeping palm of hand against door frame and elbow bent at 90 degrees, turn body from fixed hand until a stretch is felt

Cervical Spine - Lower Cervical/Upper Thoracic Stretch

- Claps hands together in front with arms extended. Gently pull shoulder blades apart and bend head forward

Chest/Biceps Stretch

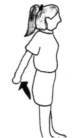

- Lace fingers behind back and squeeze shoulder blades together. Slowly raise and straighten arms

Strengthening Exercises - Biceps

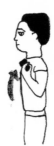

- Stand erect or sit in a chair
- Hold dumbbells at arm's length, palms in
- Keep back straight, head up, hips and legs locked
- Curl dumbbell in right hand with palm in until past thigh, then palm up for remainder of curl to shoulder
- Keep palms up while lowering until past thigh, then turn palms in
- Keep upper arms close to side
- Do a repetition with right arm, then curl left arm or do both arms at the same time

Triceps

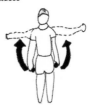

- Stand erect or sit in a chair
- Hold dumbbell in right hand; raise overhead to arm's length, upper arm close to head
- Lower dumbbell in semicircular motion behind head until forearm touches biceps
- Return to starting position and repeat with left arm

Shoulder Flexion

- Start with arm at side.
- Lift your arm toward the ceiling, keeping the arm straight

Shoulder - Progressive Resistive Exercises - Abduction (Standing)

- Raise arms out from body

Knee Lifts

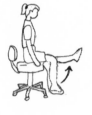

- Repeat desired number of times

Seated Knee Extension

- From a seated position, slowly straighten leg. Slowly return to start position

Knee Flexion

- Standing, bend knee up as far as possible
- Hold for 2 seconds

Hip Flexion

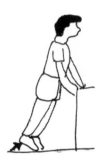

- Hip flexion with support for balance
- Hold for 2 seconds

Heel Raises

- Repeat desired number of times

Hip Extension

- Hip extension with support for balance
- Hold for 2 seconds

Hip Abduction

- Bring leg out to side
- Hold for 2 seconds

Theraband Exercises

Shoulder Flexion

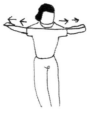

- Sit or stand on firm surface with the Theraband held at hip or waist height
- Point thumb toward ceiling. With elbow straight, raise one hand toward ceiling
- Hold. Return to start position

Chest Pull

- Sit or stand with feet shoulder width apart
- Loop the front of body with elbows slightly bent
- Pull the Theraband outwards, across chest
- Hold. Return to start position

Shoulder Extension

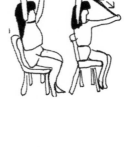

- Grasp the Theraband in palms with arm above head
- Point thumb toward ceiling. Lower arm
- Hold. Return to start position

Seated Row

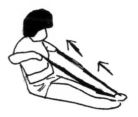

- Assume long sit position with a straight back
- With the Theraband looped under both feet, hold each end of the theraband with elbows straight
- With arms close to the sides of the body. Pull arms/elbows back
- Hold and lower slowly. Return to start position

Other Exercises Yon Can Do at Home

Shoulder Adduction

- Tie the Theraband at arm's length height
- Keep elbow straight. Pull the Theraband toward the midline of body using a sweeping motion
- Hold. Return to start position

Isometric External Rotation

- Keeping arm tucked in at side, press back of hand into wall
- Hold for 3 seconds

Hand - Towel Roll Squeeze

- With forearm resting on surface, gently squeeze towel

Supination / Pronation

- Hold your elbow bent and close to your side
- Turn your palm towards the ceiling
- Turn your palm towards the floor
- Remember to keep your elbow at your side

Back - Bilateral Scapular Retraction

- Wrap tubing around both fists
- Pull arms back while bringing shoulder blades together as if rowing a boat

Ankle and Foot - Sitting Toe Raises

- Raise toes off floor. Keep heels on floor

Sitting Heel Rise

- Rise up on balls of feet

Seated Hip Flexion

- Sit on high chair, stool or table
- Stretch band (Theraband) across thigh
- Lift hip and thigh off of table, stretching band

Hip and Knee - Resisted Hip Flexion

- With tubing around involving ankle and opposite end secured in doorjamb, bring leg forward, keeping knee straight

Resisted Hip Extension

- With tubing about involved ankle and opposite end secured in doorjamb, face door and pull leg straight back

Resisted Hip Abduction

- With tubing about involved leg and opposite end secured in doorjamb, stand sideways from door and extend leg out to the side

Wall Slides

- Leaning on wall, slowly lower buttocks toward floor until your thighs are parallel to floor. Hold for 2 seconds
- Tighten thigh muscle as you return to standing position

Back Exercises

Exercises to decrease the strain on your back

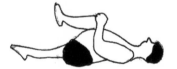

Pull one knee into chest until a comfortable stretch is felt in the lower back and buttocks. Hold for 5 seconds. Repeat 5 times with each leg.

Lie on your stomach. Raise the top half of your body as high as possible, allowing your hips and legs to remain flat on the bed. Hold

the position for 5 seconds. Repeat 5 times.

Exercises to strengthen your muscles.

Prop on elbows as high as possible. Keeping hips to the floor. Hold for 5 seconds, Repeat 5 times.

Keep knee straight and raise leg at hip. Hold for 5 seconds. Repeat 5 times.

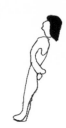

Pull both knees in to chest. Try to touch the forehead to the knees until a comfortable stretch is felt in lower back. Hold for 5 seconds, Repeat 5 times.

Stand with your feet slightly apart place your hands in the small of your back keep your knees straight. Bend backwards at the waist as far as possible and hold it for 4 seconds. Repeat 5 times.

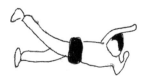

With pillow supporting abdomen, clasp hands behind back and lift upper body off floor. Hold for 5 seconds. Repeat 5 times.

Raise straight leg and opposite arm from the floor about 6 inches simultaneously. Hold for 5 seconds. Repeat 5 times

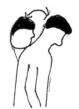

Neck Exercises

Bend your neck forward (Flexion) and backwards (extension) in full range as shown in the picture. Hold for a while, take it back to normal. Repeat 5 times.

Keep your hand as shown in the picture, rotate the shoulder both clockwise and counterclockwise and anticlockwise, take it back to normal.

Bend your neck sideways as shown in the picture. Hold it for a while. Repeat 5 times.

Elevate the shoulder as shown in the picture hold for a while bring it to normal. Repeat 5 times.

Using hand as a resistance forcing flexion & extension, hold for a while. Repeat 5 times.

Use a thin, soft pillow or dog bone pillow (shown in the picture) which you can make by removing some of the cotton stuff from the middle portion.

Yoga Exercises

Surya Namaskar (Sun Salutation) is a yoga sequence using various *asanas* (positions). Its origins lie in India where salutation to the rising sun is supposed to infuse energy into the body. The above sequence of

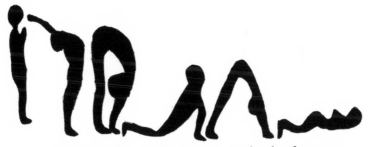

movements and *asanas* can be practiced on varying levels of awareness, ranging from that of physical exercise in various styles, to a complete sense of meditation.

Measuring Exercise Intensity

It is hard to measure how much energy you are using during the day. In an effort to quantify the energy expenditure of activities of daily living and physical exercise there are some techniques that you can utilize.

- **Talk Test:** The talk test allows you to gauge the intensity of you physical activity. At light intensity a person should be able to sing without any shortness of breath. Moderate exercise a person will be able to carry out a normal conversation. At vigorous intensity a person is too winded to carry out a normal conversation.

- **Heart rate:** If your goal is to improve the fitness of your heart and lungs, you should bring your heart rate to a range called the "target heart rate zone." When you stop exercising, quickly take your pulse to find out your heart beats per minute (see picture). Figure your maximum heart rate by subtracting your age from 220. Your target heart rate zone should be 50 to 75% of your maximum heart rate. So, if you're 50 years old, your maximum heart rate is 170 and your target heart rate zone is 85 to 127.

My target heart rate range: ....beats per minute (bpm)

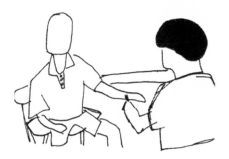

- **Perceived exertion scale:** A measurement that allows an individual to assign a numerical value to what a person is feeling in terms of physical stress and fatigue. The scale goes from 6 (at rest) to 20 (maximal exertion)

Exertion Score	Level of Exertion
6	No exertion at all
7-8	Extremely Light
9-10	Very Light
11-12	Light
13-14	Somewhat Hard
15-18	Hard (Heavy)
19	Extremely Hard
20	Maximal Exertion

- **Metabolic Equivalent of Task (MET):** or simply metabolic equivalent was created. This is a measurement expressing the energy cost of physical activities. Below is a table that represents the activities of daily living.

Table 3: Representative Levels of Energy Expenditure (in METs)

1.5 – 2 METs	4 – 5 METs
<ul><li>Walking @ 1 mph</li><li>Standing</li><li>Driving automobile</li><li>Sitting at desk or typing</li></ul>	<ul><li>Calisthenics</li><li>Cycling outdoors @ 6 mph</li><li>Golfing (carrying clubs)</li><li>Playing tennis (doubles)</li></ul>
2 – 3 METs	5 – 6 METs
<ul><li>Walking at 2.5 – 3 mph</li><li>Dusting furniture, light house work</li><li>Preparing a meal</li></ul>	<ul><li>Walking @ 4 mph</li><li>Digging in garden</li><li>Ice or roller skating @ 9 mph</li><li>Doing carpentry</li></ul>
3 – 4 METs	6 – 7 METs
<ul><li>Sweeping</li><li>Ironing</li><li>Walking 3 mph</li><li>Golfing (power cart)</li><li>Pushing light lawnmower</li></ul>	<ul><li>Stationary cycling (vigorous)</li><li>Playing Tennis (singles)</li><li>Shoveling Snow</li><li>Mowing Lawn (non-powered)</li></ul>

How can you use your energy efficiently?

Just as there are limited energy resources in the world, our bodies also have limited energy. And the same way that we are encouraged to go green by turning off lights and wasting less gasoline, you should find ways to make your own energy last longer. If we use our energy efficiently, we can accomplish more. The keys to energy efficiency are: Setting priorities, planning and pacing.

The first step is setting priorities. What are the things that need to be done on a daily, weekly, or monthly basis? Which of these things are you able to do and want to continue to do and which of these things do you do out of habit rather than need or desire? Which tasks can be done with assistance and which tasks are better delegated to someone else? Remember to include regular exercise and enjoyable leisure activities in your daily routine.

Planning will help you accomplish the task in the most efficient manner. Planning includes deciding where to do the activity, when to do it and what tools or equipment you will need.

Pacing means working at a moderate, rather than rapid rate. Pacing means alternating between heavy and light tasks and spreading strenuous activities throughout the day or the week. Pacing means taking 10 minute breaks each hour and scheduling short (20-30 minute) rests periods twice a day. Following is a listing of common activities and suggestions for using energy efficiency strategies for accomplishing them.

Coping with Breathing Problems

Once you have spoken to your doctor, you may find that following the basic advice listed below can also help manage your symptoms.

- Set your priorities. Use your energy on the things that matter most first and work down the list.
- If you can, sit down for activities such as preparing meals, shaving, or doing dishes.
- Plan ahead so that you can balance your time and energy.
- Exercise, but don't overdo it! Start slow and relaxed. A few minutes each day can make a big difference in the long run.
- Eat small, healthy meals. Not only will you keep a regular stream of nutrients and energy, but large meals take up space that your lungs could be using to breathe.
- Avoid foods that give you gas or make you constipated, as this also takes up space that your lungs could be using.
- Drinking lots of fluid can help thin phlegm. If you do cough, this will make it easier to clear your lungs and airways.

Chapter 8

Health Maintenance

*"To keep the body in good health is a duty...
otherwise we shall not be able to keep our mind
strong and clear."*

Buddha (563 BC – 483 BC)

While your doctor is providing you the best way to manage your disease medically, ultimately you are in charge of your own health. In this section, you'll find practical advice on how to handle your health and other suggestions to make life easier, healthier and more positive.

See your doctor regularly
Even if you're feeling fine, stick to your appointment schedule. Schedule your next appointment while you're at the office, so you won't forget. When you visit your physician in addition to your prescribed medications please be sure to inform them of any vitamins, herbal supplements or alternative medicines you may be taking. It is also important to notify your physician of any allergies to food or medications. Common food allergies may be to peanuts, milk, soy, nuts from trees, eggs and wheat.

Take your medications as prescribed
Bring an updated list of your medication to be reconciled with your chart on every visit. Provide your physician's with a mail order pharmacy number as well as a local pharmacy. If you are on CPAP/BiPAP/nebulizer therapy please provides your physician with a number to your durable medical equipment company. Before you leave your doctor's office make sure your refills have been ordered. You may have more than one medical condition that must be considered when making a dietary plan, so always talk with a healthcare provider or registered dietician before making changes in your diet. Set up a system that will help you remember to take your medications at the appropriate times. On the day of an appointment, schedule time in to take your medications.

Track your condition and symptoms

Prior to coming to your doctor's visit you should also write down any questions or topics you want to discuss with your doctor. In addition please keep a log of your blood pressure, sugars, oxygen saturation. Make it a point to discuss all of you current and previous lab work. Record dates of all previous diagnostic testing such as echocardiography, stress test and radiological testing.

Quit Smoking

One of the best ways you can make a positive change in your heart and lung condition is to stop smoking. (See Chapter 10). If possible, cut down on the irritants in the air where you work and live, for example, by avoiding hair spray or other aerosol sprays.

Be active and get stronger

Talk to your doctor about what activities are appropriate to do. With regular exercise, you may find an improvement in your symptoms, appetite; sleep patterns and your overall sense of well-being. Regular physical activity reduces your risk of heart disease and stroke. It also helps you reduce or control other risk factors such as high blood pressure, high blood cholesterol, excess body weight and diabetes. But the benefits don't stop there. You may look and feel better, become stronger and more flexible, have more energy and reduce stress and tension. The time to start is now.

Exercise regularly

Walking is an excellent activity. Start walking at a slow, comfortable pace for a short period of time (try 5 to 10 minutes) three to five days each week. When you're able to walk the entire time without stopping to rest, you can increase your walking duration by 1 to 2 minutes each week. A sign of a healthy lifestyle is taking 10,000 steps a day. You can monitor your steps per a day by acquiring a podometer which is available at most sporting or health store. Choose activities you enjoy. Pick a starting date that fits your schedule and gives you enough time to begin your program, like a Saturday. Some tips to help you exercise are:

- Wear comfortable clothes and shoes.
- Start slowly - don't overdo it.
- Try to exercise at the same time so it becomes a regular part of your lifestyle. For example, you might walk every day (during

your lunch hour) from 12:00 to 12:30 or start each morning with stretching and strength training.

- Drink lots of water before, during and after each exercise session.
- Ask a friend to start a program with you.
- Note the days you exercise and write down the distance or length of time of your workout and how you feel after each session. You may also want to note if your muscles are tired the next day.
- If you miss a day, plan a make-up day. Don't double your exercise time during your next session.

Conserve your energy - Though exercise is a vital part of therapy it is important to not to overexert yourself as this may actually make your breathing worse.

Have a positive attitude - Try not to compare yourself with others. Your goal should be your own personal health and fitness. Think about whether you like to exercise alone or with other people, outside or inside, what time of day is best and what kind of exercise you most enjoy doing.

- Join a support group
- Join an exercise class
- Exercise with friends or family to help motivate you.

Relax - When you feel stressed, consider a stress reduction strategy as discussed later in the chapter.

Maintain a healthy weight - Increased body weight will greater the demand on your heart and lungs. To maintain a healthy weight eat smaller portions, exercise more frequently and discuss with your doctor of medical weight loss management.

Breathe better air - It is important to stay away from cigarette smoking as well as second hand smoke, irritants, mold or any other respiratory triggers. Use an air conditioner and change the air filters frequently to keep the air less humid, cleaner and more comfortable to breathe.

Pulmonary rehabilitation - Participate in a pulmonary rehab program, as discussed previously (See Chapter 7).

Vaccinations - It is very important to stay up to date on your vaccinations. For more information on vaccination please see Chapter 4 and Appendix 3.

Stick to the plan - If you want to optimize your health, stick to your pulmonary treatment, even if it doesn't feel like it's making much of a difference right now stock to your management plan over the course of your treatment, there will be ups and downs. Don't let either success or failure of a treatment to work shake your routine. Follow your treatment plan and if you have a question, discuss it with your doctor.

Stay motivated for optimum health.

- Use a variety of exercises to keep your interest up. For example walk one day, take a swim the next and then go for a bike ride on the weekend.
- Try finding some exercise videos online. Find exercises or style of workouts you find the most interesting.
- Make exercise part of your regular routine so it becomes a habit which you become accustomed to.
- If you take a break from exercising for any length of time, don't lose hope! Just get started again, slowly and work up to your old pace.
- Don't push yourself too hard. You should be able to talk during exercise. Also, if you don't feel recovered within 10 minutes of stopping exercise, you're working too hard.
- If you have heart disease or have had a stroke, members of your family also may be at higher risk. It's very important for them to make changes now to lower their risk.

Mind Body Activities

Such activities provide a good workout, release tension and decrease anxiety while promoting health benefits. Yoga, a 5000 year old Indian practice, is one such activity and is the best-known mind-body exercise. It involves a series of sitting and laying down postures that help along with coordinated breathing and meditation techniques. Another such technique is Tai Chi, a Chinese method of slow body movement that promotes relaxation. Pilates like, yoga concentrates on breathing while strengthening the body's core muscles. Meditation can help reduce stress, anxiety and improve quality of life. It is recommended that you get involved in such activities as part of your therapy.

Stress Reduction Techniques - Relaxation and Psychophysical Techniques

The close association between dyspnea and anxiety is well known. If dyspnea is escalated and reinforced by anxiety, as many of you have experienced, a strategy must be developed to reduce the intensity and distress of dyspnea. There are a variety of different techniques that will help you relax during occasions of severe dyspnea and/or anxiety, as well as to decrease stress in daily life. Progressive muscle relaxation is a widely used technique. Some common components of most relaxation techniques include the following:

- A quiet environment
- A confortable position
- Loose, non-restrictive clothes
- Adoption of a passive attitude

Progressive Muscle Relaxation

- Close your eyes
- Perform 2 large cleansing breaths followed by your pursed-lip breathing
- With your eyes closed, try to visualize your favorite place to visit. Visualize in your mind the environment, the scenery, the smells and the colors. Try to get in touch with how you feel when you are there. Calm, relaxed and peaceful. Your breathing will begin to slow; you will take slower and deeper breaths.
- Perform slow abdominal breathing with a deep inhalation and a slow exhalation through pursed lips.
- Optional: follow the above mentioned steps followed by systematic tensing then relaxing every part of the body including feet, arms, legs, chest, face, eyes, shoulders, etc., concentrating on each muscle as the tension and relaxation is performed.

The ABC's of Better Breathing

- **A**lways be positive! – Each day is a new day and you can make an effort to improve your breathing.
- **B**reathe – Your breathing is something that can be improved with a little work and exercise. Follow the guidance of your physician and rehab counselors.
- **C**oncentrate – Hone in on the process of breathing so you can gain a better understanding of it and how to control it better.
- **D**iary – Keep a diary of things that made your breathing worse or techniques you used to make it better
- **E**xhale - During any activity in which you have to exert yourself don't forget to exhale. Exhaling as much as you can will help make your breathing more efficient.
- **F**ollow - Your doctor's recommendations may be the key to your breathing success. Be sure to take all the medications and follow all instructions your doctor has suggested to you. These recommendations will help maintain your overall and pulmonary well-being.
- **G**row – Advanced lung disease is a chronic condition. You will have to grow with it and learn to control it, not let it control you.
- **H**elp – Don't be afraid to ask for help when a task is difficult or overwhelming. Seek help in understanding your illness or aspects of your care
- **I**nhale - Make sure to inhale when you are involved in active motion. This allows for maximum amount of oxygenation of the blood that is being returned from your body.
- **J**ump - Jump to action! If you notice any changes in your breathing alert your physician immediately. These symptoms may be due to a treatable cause.
- **K**eep calm - When you feel anxious or an episode of shortness of breath coming on stay calm and focus on your breathing. Remember the breathing exercises that were taught to you by your physician or respiratory therapist.
- **L**ive efficiently - Live each day to its fullest! Just because you are faced with a chronic illness does not mean you should stop enjoying your life and things you like to do (although some activities may need to be done in moderation)
- **M**anage your medications! Keep a log of what medications you are taking, who prescribed them and why.

- **N**ever leave the house without your inhalers and a list of all your medications. This could be vital information that may become necessary shall an emergency arise.
- **O**xygenate - If you're breathing is becoming a handicap, then talk to your physician about oxygen therapy.
- **P**ace – Pace yourself. When at home, there is no need to rush. Complete all household tasks at your own pace. This will prevent you from getting short of breath and possible other complications.
- **Q**uit smoking - If you smoke and currently have a breathing problem, you must quit smoking. Breathing efficiency and quality starts improving from the time you put out your last cigarette.
- **R**emember – Remember your support system. Your support system is made up of your family, caregivers, physicians, respiratory therapist and anyone else that is involved in your healthcare. If you need any help with your healthy remember to contact the appropriate individual without delay.
- **S**upport groups – There exists, a support group for virtually all pulmonary diseases. Please, with the aid of your physician discover what support groups pertain to you. There is a vast amount of resources available to help you with your condition as well as your breathing like the Pulmonary Hypertension Association (www.PHAssociation.org) and the Pulmonary Fibrosis Foundation (www.pulmonaryfibrosis.org).
- **T**ake – It's important that you take all your medications as your doctor has prescribed them. Take advice. All of your healthcare providers are there to help you. It is also important NOT to stop any medication without consulting a health care provider.
- **U**nderstanding your disease – You have to be proactive. Taking an active approach to your health is the best way you can help your breathing. Becoming educated on your own medical condition will help you better understand the cause of your breathing problems and in turn help you manage it.
- **V**entilation – It's important to keep the air in your house well ventilated and in constant circulation. Smoke, steam, dust, pets and other irritants may worsen your breathing. Ask your physician about proper ventilation methods.
- **W**atch for breathing pitfalls – Breathing pitfalls are situations in which you arrive that will cost you lots of energy. For example,

forgetting something on the first floor when you come upstairs. This would require you to make an extra trip

- **eX**ercise - Slow but steady physical and strength training exercises can help you better your breathing efficiency. It may be difficult at first but it will eventually help your breathing.
- **Y**esterday is gone! Focus on what you can do today to improve your health & well being.
- **Z**est – Incorporate some activities in your life that make you happy. Being in a better mood can increase your overall health; help improve you breathing and outlook on life.

Positive Emotion Through Life Skills Training

Appreciate what you already have.

- Once a week write down 5 things that you are thankful for.
- Give thanks for your food and be mindful when you eat.
- Remind yourself of the gift of each new breath.
- Appreciate the beauty in nature.
- Call up people to say thank you for their friendship or care.
- Remember that nothing is guaranteed and nothing lasts forever.
- Look for the good in people.
- Learn to Relax, slow down and do one thing at a time, Slow and deep diaphragmatic breathing.
- Use a mantra.

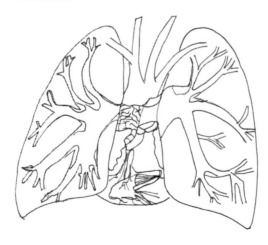

Respond appropriately to disappointment.

- Understand that everyone will be disappointed at times. Be prepared by realizing some things will never change. Learn what these are and find the best way for you to work around them.
- All frustrations spring from not getting what you want. Ask yourself if you can control the situation. Don't worry about things that you cannot change.
- Practice forgiveness. Ask yourself, "What am I already doing to solve the problem that does not work.
- You are not alone. Remember that there are many people who have struggled with the same problems you have.

How can visits with your primary care doctor be helpful?

Visit with your primary care physician are an important part of staying healthy. Many health problems that develop later on in life may be preventive by taking care of your health and keep regular checkups. Physical examination by your primary care physician and routine blood work promotes early detection of the most common yet treatable diseases, such as cancer, diabetes and heart disease.

- Well Visits for Healthy Young Adults (Ages 19-39) should be every 5 years.
- Well Visits for Healthy Adults (Ages 40-49) should be every 1 to 3 years.
- Well Visits for Adults (Ages 50 and Up) should be every 1 to 2 years

Blood tests that your primary care physician may order

Complete Blood Count (CBC)

The CBC is a test that is ordered to get a profile of the blood cells in your body. The CBC provides information about the white blood cells (WBC), the red blood cell (RBC) and platelets that are in the blood. This information includes the number, type, size, shape and some of the observations of the cells.

- White blood cells (WBC's) protect the body against infection

- Red blood cells (RBC's) carry oxygen
- Platelets help stop bleeding

Lipid Panel (Cholesterol Test)

The Cholesterol test or sometimes called the lipid test, is used to estimate your risk of developing heart disease. Cholesterol is important for your body to produce hormones and help with digestion (The breakdown of food you eat). The fats you eat are stored in the liver and travel through the body along with Cholesterol. Cholesterol particles are made up of proteins and fats that are bound together to form three main types of cholesterol. The Cholesterol test provides information on Low Density Lipoproteins (LDL), High Density Lipoproteins (HDL), Very Low Density Lipoproteins (VLDL) and Triglycerides. LDL is sticky and will stick to your arteries (Arteries are tubes that carries blood through your body, like pipes carry water to parts of your home). Target cholesterol goals are as follows: An LDL of <100 mg/dL, HDL of >40 mg/dL - and Triglycerides <150 mg/dL

- VLDL carries your triglycerides (Fats) to your fat cells.
- LDL is what remains after the fat has been delivered to its destination
- HDL carries the remaining LDL back to the liver.
- Triglycerides are fats in your blood used to store energy when needed.

Glucose Testing

To correctly assess the sugar level in your body a basic metabolic panel may be ordered to get an idea of a random glucose level. However to better gauge how the sugar levels have been running in the body for the last 8-10 weeks your physician may order a test, called the glycosylated hemoglobin (HemoglobinA1C). The A1C test is a blood test that measure how much sugar is attached to the hemoglobin protein that is present inside your red blood cells. It is important that your HgbA1C be checked routinely every 6 months and every 3-6 months for diabetics. The target glucose goal should be a glucose of <100 mg/dL and a hemoglobinA1C of 3.5%-5.5%.

Diabetes occurs when your body is unable to handle the amount of sugars in your blood. Insulin (A hormone made by the pancreas) moves sugars in your blood to your cells. Your cells use the sugars as fuel for energy. If you have too much sugar in your blood, your cells become non respondent to insulin's request to your cells to process sugar.

Comprehensive Metabolic Panel (CMP)

The CMP is routinely ordered as part of a blood work-up for a medical exam or your yearly physical. The test is usually conducted after you have been fasting. This test will test the electrolytes in your body as well as the liver and kidney function. These test may not tell you physician what exactly what is wrong with you but may give an idea of what may be causing the abnormal test results.

Kidney Tests

- **BUN (blood urea nitrogen) and Creatinine**

Urea is the waste product of your body after your body uses proteins. Urea is sent from your kidneys and cleared by your body as urine. Creatinine is a waste product in the formation of muscle. These tests are used to see how well your kidneys are removing waste in your body.

The estimated glomerular filtration rate (eGFR) is a calculation used to see how well your kidneys are working. Kidney disease is best treated when diagnosed in its early stages.

Table 4: Stages of Kidney Disease

Kidney Damage Stage	Description	GFR	Other findings
1	Kidney damage with normal or high GFR	90+	Protein or albumin in urine are high, cells or casts seen in urine
2	Mild decrease in GFR	60-89	
3	Moderate decrease in GFR	30-59	
4	Severe decrease in GFR	15-29	
5	Kidney failure	< 15	

Liver Tests

- ALP (alkaline phosphatase)
- ALT (alanine amino transferase, also called SGPT)
- AST (aspartate amino transferase, also called SGOT)
- Bilirubin

ALP, ALT and AST are enzymes found in the liver and other tissues. These enzymes are used to determine if your liver is working properly. Bilirubin is a waste product when your liver eliminates old red blood cells.

Other Regular Health Maintenance Testing

- Blood Pressure monitoring and measurement every few months
- Colonoscopy every 5 years
- Eye exam every 2 years (Every one year for Diabetics)
- For women, a pap smear periodically as recommended by OB/GYN.
- For males Prostate Specific Antigen (PSA) every year.

Chapter 9

<u>Lung Disease & Other Health</u>
<u>Problems</u>

"The good physician treats the disease; the great physician treats the patient who has the disease."

Sir William Osler (1849-1919)

Osteoporosis and Lung Disease

Bone is composed of bone cells, collagen, calcium and phosphorus. Bone accrual occurs steadily through childhood and 40%-50% of bone mineral accrual occurs during the teenage years into the early twenties. During this process bone is built, bone is broken down and bone is rebuilt to improve the strength of bone. The majority of this bone accrual is determined by genetics, but factors such as diet and exercise contribute. With aging, the amount of bone that is broken down exceeds the amount of bone that is built and individuals whose bone accrual during the teenage years is sub-optimal are at increased risk for osteoporosis later in life. However, pulmonary patients (both male and female) are often at higher risk for losing bone mass, especially those with more advanced disease.

Osteoporosis can also negatively affect the lungs as it progresses. When bones begin to lose their mass, they are prone to fractures, including compression and fragility fractures. Fractures that occur in the vertebrae (spine), hip and ribs can be particularly problematic. These pathologic fractures lead to decrease of mobility. Fractures in the spine may lead to a hunching effect called kyphosis. Kyphosis restricts the expanding of the lungs which may worsen or exacerbate lung disease.

Having lung disease can put you at risk, of osteoporosis and you should discuss with your doctor how to prevent bone loss. This means getting a bone density test, ensuring that you have enough calcium and vitamin D in your diet. Make sure that you are getting rechecked as often as your doctor recommends, especially if you are taking prednisone or other steroids. Prevention of osteoporosis and maintaining healthy bones can be a great asset in your fight against lung disease.

Risk Factors for Osteoporosis:

- Glucocorticoids (e.g. prednisone, etc.) decrease bone formation
- Age related decreased in sex hormones leads to bone loss
- Poor nutrition and malabsorption can lead to deficiencies in vitamins and minerals important for the bones (D, K, Zinc, Ca).
- Lack of exercise and decreased weight-bearing activity leads to decreased muscle mass.
- Inflammation can also increase bone loss
- Renal disease can increase bone loss

Individuals with advanced lung disease will require serial DEXA evaluations depending on their bone mineral density (BMD) score. If the DEXA is normal (BMD > T -1) then the DEXA can be repeated in five years (sooner if concerns arise). If the BMD T score is between -1 and -2 the DEXA can be repeated every 2-4 years (again, sooner if concerns arise). A yearly DEXA is recommended for BMD T score of less than -2.

Prevention of poor bone health focuses on overall good nutrition, adequate supplementation of calcium, vitamin D and other vitamins and minerals, regular weight bearing exercise and avoiding excessive glucocorticoid use if possible.

Treatment is indicated for individuals who have a BMD T score of < -2. For individual's whose BMD T-score is between -1 and -2, treatment should be considered if the individual has had what is referred to as a fragility fracture (spine, rib), or if excessive loss has occurred.

Treatment options for osteoporosis in the elderly have expanded over the past few years. Biphosphonates are the mainstay of therapy. These medications prevent bone loss. Zolendronic Acid (delivered intravenously) and oral bisphosphonates increase bone mineral density and appear to decrease fracture risk in adults. Other options, for steroid induced osteoporosis, include teriparatide (Forteo®)

In the otherwise healthy population, increasing treatment strategies are becoming available to prevent and treat osteoporosis in the elderly. As individuals with advance lung disease age menopause and senile osteoporosis are additional realities, the role of bone preservation in childhood and early adult years becomes even more relevant.

Sleep Disorders

The human body needs sleep for recovery and restitution. It is an active state essential for mental and physical restoration. Regular inability to get a good night's sleep may be indicative of a sleep disorder.

Obstructive Sleep Apnea (OSA)

Obstructive Sleep Apnea is the most common sleep disorder. It is a serious and potentially life-threatening condition that often goes undiagnosed. Loud snoring may signal that something is wrong with breathing during sleep and reflect presence of OSA. The condition affects at least 2-4% of middle-aged adults. Approximately 95% of the affected population remains undiagnosed and untreated.

Some of the warning signs of OSA are, but not limited to excessive daytime fatigue and sleepiness, snoring, falling asleep at inappropriate times, poor performance at home or at work and cessation of breathing at night.

What are the Consequences of Untreated OSA?

When OSA goes untreated it may lead to elevations in blood pressure, heart arrhythmias or even heart failure, poor oxygenation, heart attack, cardiovascular accidents such as stroke. Excessive daytime sleepiness and fatigue may lead to traffic and industrial accidents.

How can Obstructive Sleep Apnea be Treated?

Currently there are a few options for the treatment of OSA. . The most effective option is a continuous positive air pressure (CPAP) machine which uses air to help keep your airways open while you sleep. Those who are intolerant to the CPAP device may be considered for surgery or an oro-dental device. The most conservative treatment option is weight loss in conjunction with lifestyle modification. You are encouraged to discuss these therapeutic options with your physician if you suspect you may have OSA symptoms or you have been diagnosed to have OSA.

How can you measure your daytime sleepiness symptoms?

Johns et al. from Australia devised a screening questionnaire called the Epworth Sleepiness Scale Score to gauge daytime sleepiness. It is a set of questions that assesses your likelihood of falling asleep during daytime situations.

Epworth Sleepiness Scale Score:

0 = Would never doze off
1 = Slight chance of dozing off
2 = Moderate chance of dozing off
3 = High chance of dozing off

_____ Sitting and reading
_____ Watching television
_____ Sitting, inactive in a public place (i.e., movie theater)
_____ Sitting talking to someone
_____ As a passenger in a car for an hour without a break
_____ Sitting quietly after lunch without alcohol
_____ Lying down to rest in the afternoon if time permitted
_____ In a car, while stopped for a few minutes in traffic
_____ **Total Score**

Johns MW. A new method for measuring daytime sleepiness: the Epworth sleepiness scale. Sleep. 1991 Dec; 14(6):540-5.

If your total score is higher than 10, it may indicate excessive daytime sleepiness which is a sign of possible OSA. You should discuss this with your physician to determine whether you may have a sleep disorder. Based on this simple questionnaire a health care provider such as a pulmonologist can better gauge if you are a candidate for a sleep study

Another questionnaire to help you gauge the likelihood of you having OSA is the STOP-Bang Questionnaire. This predicts presence of sleep apnea. Answering Yes to 3 or more questions in this questionnaire indicates high probability of presence of OSA.

STOP - Bang Scoring Model

1. Snoring
Do you snore loudly (loud enough to be heard through closed doors)?
Yes   No

2. Tired
Do you often feel tired, fatigued or sleepy during daytime?
                    Yes   No
3. Observed
Has anyone observed you stopping breathing during your sleep?
                    Yes   No
4. Blood pressure
Do you have or are you being treated for high blood pressure?
                    Yes   No
5. BMI
BMI more than 35kg/m^2?
                    Yes   No
6. Age
Age over 50 years old?
                    Yes   No
7. Neck circumference
Neck circumference greater than 40?
                    Yes   No
8. Gender
Gender male?
                    Yes   No

Chung, F., Yegneswaran, B., Liao, P., Chung, S. A., Vairavanathan, S., Islam, S., Khajehdehi, A. and Shapiro, C. M. STOP Questionnaire A Tool to Screen Obstructive Sleep Apnea. Anesthesiology 108, 812-821. 2008.

Sleep Hygiene

Poor sleep habits (referred to as hygiene) are among the most common problems encountered in our society. We stay up too late and get up too early. We interrupt our sleep with drugs, chemicals and work and we over-stimulate ourselves with late-night activities such as television. Below are some essentials of good sleep habits. Many of these points will seem like common sense. But it is surprising how many of these important points are ignored by many of us.

Your Personal Habits

- Fix a bedtime and an awakening time. Do not be one of those people who allow bedtime and awakening time to drift. The body "gets used" to falling asleep at a certain time, but only if this is relatively fixed. Even if you are retired or not working, this is an essential component of good sleeping habits.

- Avoid napping during the day. If you nap throughout the day, it is no wonder that you will not be able to sleep at night. The late afternoon for most people is a "sleepy time". Many people will take a nap at that time. This is generally not a bad thing to do, provided you limit the nap to 30-40 minutes and can sleep well at night.

- Avoid alcohol 4-6 hours before bedtime. Many people believe that alcohol helps them sleep. While alcohol has an immediate sleep-inducing effect, a few hours later as the alcohol levels in your blood start to fall, there is a stimulant or wake-up effect.

- Avoid caffeine 4-6 hours before bedtime. This includes caffeinated beverages such as coffee, tea and many sodas, as well as chocolate, so be careful. Avoid heavy, spicy, or sugary foods 4-6 hours before bedtime. These can affect your ability to stay asleep. Exercise regularly, but not right before you go to bed. Regular exercise, particularly in the afternoon, can help deepen sleep. Strenuous exercise within the 2 hours before bedtime, however, can decrease your ability to fall asleep.

- Exercise a digital curfew. Ban digital devices from the bedroom. Technology can alienate people. As smart phones continue to burrow their way into our lives, wearable devices such as Google Glass® threaten to invade out personal space even further. Draw

- a gadget free line in the bedroom. Don't sleep with your cellphone, leave it downstairs or in the living room overnight.

Your Sleeping Environment

- Use comfortable bedding. Uncomfortable bedding can prevent good sleep. Evaluate whether or not this is a source of your problem and make appropriate changes.
- Find a comfortable temperature setting for sleeping and keep the room well ventilated. If your bedroom is too cold or too hot, it can keep you awake. A cool (not cold) bedroom is often the most conducive to sleep.
- Reserve the bed for sleep. Don't use the bed as an office, workroom or recreation room. Let your body know that the bed is associated with sleeping.

Getting Ready For Bed

- **Eat Light:** Try a light snack before bed. Warm milk and foods high in the amino acid tryptophan, such as bananas, may help you to sleep.
- **Develop a Routine:** Practice relaxation techniques before bed. Relaxation techniques such as yoga, deep breathing and other may help relieve anxiety and reduce muscle tension.
- **Keep a To Do List:** Don't take your worries to bed. Leave your worries about job, school, daily life, etc., behind when you go to bed. Some people find it useful to assign a "worry period" during the evening or late afternoon to deal with these issues.
- **Establish a Pre-sleep Ritual:** Pre-sleep rituals, such as a warm bath or a few minutes of reading, can help you sleep.
- **Find a Sleeping Position:** If you don't fall asleep within 15-30 minutes, get up, go into another room and read until sleepy.
- **Power Down:** Any device with a screen (TV, tablet PC, laptop, iPad) emits a blue spectrum light that can inhibit the brain production of melatonin that induces sleep. Some people find that the radio helps them go to sleep. Since radio is a less engaging medium than TV, this might be a better idea.

Getting Up in the Middle of the Night

Most people wake up one or two times a night for various reasons. If you find that you get up in the middle of night and cannot get back to sleep within 15-20 minutes, then do not remain in the bed "trying hard" to sleep. Get out of bed, leave the bedroom, read, have a light snack, do some quiet activity or take a bath. You will generally find that you can get back to sleep 20 minutes or so later. Do not perform challenging or engaging activity such as office work, housework, etc. Do not watch television.

A Word About Sleeping Aids

Sometimes you may not have any sleep disorder but may find it hard to fall asleep. Make it a point to discuss with your physicians about sleeping aids. Common supplements for sleeping are Valerian root, melatonin and ashwagandha root. Pharmaceutical options for sleeping aids are zolpidem (Ambien®), eszopiclone (Lunesta®), zaleplon (Sonata®) or ramelteon (Rozerem®) also may help you get to sleep. Please discuss with your physician.

Obesity

Obesity has recently been recognized by the American Medical Association as a diseased state. Inactivity and a sedentary lifestyle due to lung disease may contribute to obesity. Obesity is measure in terms of body mass index (BMI) that is defined as you weight in kilograms divided by you height in meters squared. Below you will find a chart that summarizes the severity of obesity.

Where you carry your body weight also makes a difference. Excess abdominal fat (central or visceral obesity), which is found above the waist, is related to increased risk of diabetes and heart disease. In men a waist greater than 40 inches and in women more than 36 inches is of concern. While fat that accumulates under the skin or in area of hips and thighs poses less of health risks.

The following chart illustrates what that number means:

Table 5: Definition of Body Mass Index (BMI)

Body Mass Index (BMI)	Classification	What It Means
Less than 18.5	Underweight	Increased risk of health problems associated with underweight, such as inadequate nutrition.
18.5-24.9	Normal	Healthy body weight for height.
25-29.9	Overweight	Heavier than the optimal for height—carries an increased risk of weight-related health problems.
30-34.9	Obesity I	High risk of common medical problems associated with obesity, such as type 2 diabetes, high blood pressure, abnormal cholesterol and breathing disorders. In most people, a BMI of 30 means they're about 30 to 40 pounds overweight.
35-39.9	Obesity II	Very high risk of common medical problems associated with obesity such as type 2 diabetes, high blood pressure, abnormal cholesterol and breathing disorders.
40 or greater	Obesity III (severe obesity; previously referred to as morbid obesity).	Extremely high risk of associated medical problems. People with a BMI of 40 or greater are typically 100 pounds overweight or more.

Table 6: Risk level associated with waist circumference

	Risk Level	
Category	Healthy	High
Men	≤ 40"	> 40"
Women	≤ 35"	>35"

Management of obesity is centered on weight loss. There are a few options on how to approach this. The first is lifestyle modification that entails changing diet and incorporating exercise into your daily routine. There needs to be a reduction in the net calories that you're consuming to begin weight loss. In cases where lifestyle modification does not help there are pharmaceutical interventions that may kick start your metabolism. These drugs are phentermine/topiramate (Qsymia®), locaserin (Belviq®) and tetrahydrolipstatin (Orlistat®) which work suppressing appetite. For a select few patients where the above two options do not work surgical intervention may be necessary. Please consult with your physician regarding your weight loss options.

Metabolic Syndrome

Metabolic syndrome is a condition defined as a cluster of three or more of the following risk factors in adults:

- Increased abdominal fat: waist circumference in a woman of at least 35 inches, or 40 inches or greater in a man
- Elevated blood pressure on several measurements: 130 or greater systolic (top number) or 85 or greater diastolic (bottom number)
- Elevated level of triglycerides (blood fats): greater than 150 after a twelve-hour fast
- Low level of high-density lipoprotein (HDL)- the "good" cholesterol: under 40 for a man or less than 50 for a woman
- Elevated blood sugar: 110 or greater after a twelve-hour fast—for instance, first thing in the morning, before breakfast; this includes blood sugars in the pre-diabetes range

If you have metabolic syndrome, you face an increased chance of developing cholesterol deposits in the arterial walls (*atherosclerosis*), which causes most heart attacks and strokes and also an increased risk for developing diabetes. Metabolic syndrome occurs in only 5 percent of adults of normal weight, but in 22 percent of those who are overweight and in 60 percent of those who are obese! For these people, the most important interventions are weight loss and exercise.

High blood pressure (Hypertension)

Blood pressure is the force of blood pushing against the inside of your blood vessels, called arteries, as your heart pumps. High blood pressure is a serious condition that causes your heart to work harder. It is also called hypertension. It can cause heart disease, stroke, kidney failure, blood vessel disease and other health problems. Those who are more likely to have high blood pressure include:

- African Americans
- Men over the age of 45 and women over the age of 55
- People with a family history of high blood pressure
- Women who are pregnant, or who take birth control pills, or hormone replacement therapy
- People with health conditions like thyroid disease, chronic kidney disease, or sleep apnea
- Those who take certain medicines, such as asthma medicines and cold-relief products

Your chances of having high blood pressure increase if you:

- Are overweight
- Eat foods high in salt
- Do not get regular exercise
- Smoke
- Drink alcohol heavily

There is no way to tell that you have high blood pressure. The only way to know if you have high blood pressure is to have it checked. The following are some key points regarding your blood pressure measurement:

- There are two blood pressure numbers. Systolic (top number) - the pressure when your heart pumps the blood out of your body.
- Diastolic (bottom number) - the pressure when your heart is resting in between beats.
- Your blood pressure should be less than 120/80 mmHg. (120 is your systolic number, 80 is your diastolic number)
- High blood pressure is when your blood pressure is 140/90 mmHg or greater.
- "Pre-hypertension" is when your blood pressure is greater than 120/ 80 mmHg, but less than 140/90 mmHg. When you have pre-hypertension, you may be at risk for high blood pressure and other health related problems.
- If you have diabetes or kidney problems, your blood pressure should be less than 130/80 mmHg.

What changes can I make in my life if I have high blood pressure?

High blood pressure needs to be controlled. You can change or control some lifestyle habits that will help treat, prevent or delay high blood pressure. These include:

- healthy eating - choosing a low salt or no salt diet
- staying physically active
- keeping or getting to a healthy weight
- quitting smoking
- limiting alcoholic drinks to 1-2 a day
- dealing with stress in a healthy way
- taking your high blood pressure medicine as prescribed
- keeping all appointments with your doctor

What should I do if I have high blood pressure?

If you have high blood pressure, you should:

- Know your blood pressure numbers, write them down and keep a record.
- Ask your doctor about a home blood pressure monitoring kit and what you need to do to help lower your blood pressure.

Heart Disease and Stroke

There are many types of heart and blood vessel diseases. Each year more than 870,000 people die from them. Here are some key steps you can take:

- Don't smoke and avoid other people's tobacco smoke.
- Be physically active
- Keep your weight under control
- Get regular medical check ups
- Eat a healthy diet low in saturated fat, cholesterol and salt.
- Control your blood sugar if you have diabetes

Hardening of the arteries or atherosclerosis is when the inner walls of arteries become narrower due to a buildup of plaque. This limits the flow of blood to the heart and brain. Sometimes this plaque can break open. When this happens, a blood clot forms and blocks the artery. This can cause heart attacks and strokes.

Heart attacks occur when the blood flow to a part of the heart is blocked, usually by a blood clot. If this clot cuts off the blood flow completely, the part of the heart muscle supplied by that artery begins to die. Here are some of the signs that can mean a heart attack is happening:

- Uncomfortable pressure, squeezing, fullness or pain in the center of your chest. It lasts more than a few minutes, or goes away and comes back.
- Pain or discomfort in one or both arms.
- Shortness of breath with or without chest discomfort.
- Other signs such as breaking out in a cold sweat, nausea or lightheadedness.

If you have one or more of these signs, don't wait more than 5 minutes before calling for help. Call 9-1-1. Get to a hospital right away.

Strokes and Transient Ischemic Attacks (TIA - "mini-stroke") happen when a blood vessel that feeds the brain gets clogged or bursts. Then that part of the brain can't work and neither can the part of the body it controls. Major causes of stroke include:

- High blood pressure
- Smoking
- Diabetes
- High cholesterol
- Heart disease
- Atrial fibrillation (Abnormal heart rhythm)

There are some imaging tests that may be used to help determine your risk for possible heart attack or stroke: (Please refer to Chapter 3)

- Stroke/carotid artery ultrasound – a test used to measure blockages in the arteries that supply the brain. This test is recommended for people with risk factors for vascular disease like hypertension

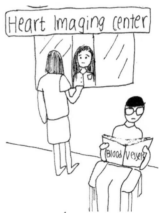

Call 9-1-1 to get help fast if you have any of these warning signs of stroke and TIA:

- Sudden numbness or weakness of the face, arm or leg, especially on one side of the body
- Sudden confusion, trouble speaking or understanding
- Sudden trouble seeing in one or both eyes
- Sudden trouble walking, dizziness, loss of balance or coordination
- Sudden, severe headache with no known cause

Diabetes

Diabetes is defined as increased sugar levels in the bloodstream. There are two types of diabetes, Type 1 (autoimmune destruction of the pancreas) and Type 2 that is linked with obesity and insulin resistance. A diagnosis of diabetes is made when you have a fasting sugar level of 126 or higher on two or more occasions or a HemoglobinA1C level of more than 6.5%. Recommended levels of blood glucose before a meal (pre-prandial) are 70–125 mg/dl (5.0–7.2 mmol/l). After a meal (postprandial) the sugars should be less than 180 mg/dl (Less than 10.0 mmol/l)

Blood sugar levels rise and fall throughout the day. By checking your blood sugar you can learn how well your diabetes care plan is working. Understanding why your blood glucose changes can help you to keep your blood glucose on target.

- Eat a well balanced diet as outlined by your nutritionist. A healthy diet for a person with diabetes is a healthy diet for everyone. Avoid foods that are high in fats and simple carbohydrates. Foods to avoid include fruit juices, bagels, pizza and fast food.
- If you have no contraindications (ulcer, bleeding tendency, other blood thinners, etc) take a regular or coated aspirin every day.
- You should have your A1C tested every three months. This test tells how well you've controlled your blood sugar during the past 3 months. An A1C of less than 6.8% is recommended.
- Make sure you know your cholesterol level and have it checked every year. Your LDL or bad cholesterol should be below 100 mg/dl. Your HDL or good cholesterol should be above 40 mg/dl. Your triglycerides should be below 150 mg/dl.
- Keep your blood pressure below 130/80. This will help to keep your heart, kidneys and eyes healthy.
- People with diabetes must see an ophthalmologist for a yearly eye exam. Make sure you tell your eye doctor that you have diabetes.
- You should have a urine test for "microalbumin" (tiny amounts of protein) at least once a year.
- Try to include exercise in your daily routine. You should be exercising at least 30 minutes each day unless otherwise advised.
- Smoking is extremely dangerous for people with diabetes. There are many tools available to help you quit.
- Be sure to get the influenza vaccine every year.

Write down all blood glucose results in a log or record book. Bring them with you to all of your appointments. Your results will help you and your healthcare team will make decisions about your diabetes treatment plan. For a list of diabetes medications please refer to Appendix 4

Obesity Hypoventilation Syndrome (OHS)

As most people already know, how much you weigh plays a big impact on your health in general. In addition, persons with chronic lung disease are often sedentary, which can lead to weight gain. Being overweight has an effect on many of the body's systems and organs, which then has an indirect effect on the lungs. The measurement of obesity is made using the body mass index (BMI) scale which is explained above.

Obesity Hypoventilation syndrome is a disorder that is characterized by the concomitant existence of obesity, increase levels of daytime carbon dioxide in the blood and sleep disordered breathing. This may be seen in the setting of OSA that was explained above. The mechanism by which this disorder develops is thought to be due to the fat deposits in the chest that has a mechanical effect on making breathing more difficult. A person's body mass index (BMI) and abdominal fat are more relevant in obesity hypoventilation syndrome.

Sleep disordered breathing such at Obstructive Sleep Apnea is also common in people who have OHS. This combined with higher levels of carbon dioxide in the blood during the daytime can make a person feel excessively tired. Too much carbon dioxide in the blood can also have more serious consequences, such as a lower level of consciousness or abnormal blood acidity, both of which can require hospitalization.

The only truly effective treatment for OHS is weight loss. This may be achieved either through diet and exercise, or in extreme cases, bariatric surgery. Both methods of weight loss have a positive effect on OHS symptoms. However, patients that incorporate exercise into their weight loss will also receive the therapeutic benefits of exercise on the lungs. In some cases, your doctor may prescribe a CPAP machine, which will help keep your airways open while you sleep. While this may help to alleviate some symptoms, OHS can only be reversed by weight loss.

Kidneys and Lung Disease

The kidneys are organs in your body that have a lot of important function. These include getting rid of all waste products via making of urine. The kidneys are powerful set of organs that perform the following functions:

- Remove waste products from the body
- Remove drugs and toxins from the body
- Balances the electrolytes in your body
- Regulates blood pressure
- Regulates Vitamin D production
- Regulates your hemoglobin count and prevents from anemia

The kidneys work hand in hand with your heart and lungs to regulate the body's function. In the setting of advanced lung disease the kidneys may be starved of necessary oxygen. When the lungs are not able to properly oxygenate the blood it's called hypoxemia which will ultimately cause the kidney to not function properly.

What happens when kidneys don't work?

- You are unable to get rid of your waste products and toxins build up and as a result you feel fatigue, weakness, tremors, decreased urine output are symptoms of kidney disease.
- You are unable to regulate blood pressure and fluid, resulting in hypertension or elevated blood pressure.
- If you cannot make the hormone for red blood cells, you get anemic or your hemoglobin amount drops.
- If you cannot make vitamin D, it leads to bone loss.
- You get puffiness around your eyes, hands and feet
- Your blood pressure on physical exam can be elevated.

How is Kidney Disease Detected?

Early detection and treatment of chronic kidney disease are extremely important for prevention of kidney problems. 3 simple tests can help tremendously.

- A test for protein and blood in the urine. This can be obtained by giving a urine sample to your doctor and getting a urinalysis done. When there is injury to the filtering unit of the kidney, the kidneys start losing protein and blood in the urine and you can only notice this microscopically.
- A test for blood creatinine. Your doctor should use your results, along with your age, race, gender and other factors, to calculate your glomerular filtration rate (GFR). Your GFR tells how much kidney function you have.
- An elevated blood pressure can be an earlier sign of kidney disease.

If you suffer from advance lung disease please ask your physicians about your kidney function. They may refer you for some laboratory testing or even to a specialist to have your kidneys evaluated.

Chapter 10

Lungs and Tobacco

"Smoking is hateful to the nose, harmful to the brain and dangerous to the lungs."

King James I (1566-1625)

By now, you are well aware that smoking damages your lungs. If you smoke, quitting is the number one thing that you can do to improve your standard of living, more than diet, exercise, medications, or rehab. It is important to note that no matter how severe your lung disease is smoking decreases quality of life. If you do not smoke, but someone in your household does, even if they don't smoke inside, you may be at increased risk of smoke-related problems. Even today Tobacco use is the second cause of death globally (after high blood pressure) and is currently responsible for killing one in ten adults worldwide. Below are facts about smoking, which illustrate just how important it is for someone with any stage of disease to kick the habit.

How do I know how addicted I am to cigarettes?

Most people who smoke will be able to tell you how many cigarettes they smoke in a day. They may also be able to tell how addicted they are to smoking. Below you will find a simple scale to assess how much you are addicted to cigarettes.

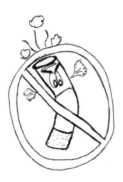

Fagerström Nicotine Dependence Scale

	0	1	2	3
How soon after you wake up do you smoke your first cigarette?	After 60 minutes	31-60 Minutes	6-30 Minutes	Within 5 minutes
Do you find it difficult to refrain from smoking in places where it is forbidden, e.g., in church, at the library, cinema, etc?	No	Yes		
Which cigarette would you hate most to give up?	All Others	First one in the morning		
How many cigarettes/day do you smoke?	10 or less	11-20	21-30	31 or more
Do you smoke more frequently during the first hours of waking than during the rest of the day?	No	Yes		
Do you smoke if you are so ill that you are in bed most of the day?	No	Yes		

Heatherton TF, Kozlowski LT, Frecker RC, Fagerström KO. The Fagerström Test for Nicotine Dependence: a revision of the Fagerström Tolerance Questionnaire. Br J Addict. 1991 Sep;86(9):1119-27.

Scoring of Fagerström Nicotine Dependency Scale

Three yes/no items are scored 0 (no) and 1 (yes). The 3 multiple-choice items are scored from 0 to 3.

0-2	Very Low Dependence
3-4	Low Dependence
5	Moderate Dependence
6-7	High Dependence
8-10	Very High Dependence

What does smoking do to my lungs?

Damages the airways

- Your airways will become inflamed.
- The little hair like structures, called cilia, that usually move back and forth to sweep particles out of the airways will stop working normally. Cilia in the airways move particles cephalad and are paralyzed by tobacco smoke.
- Your large airways will produce more mucus, which can cause a chronic cough. This is called chronic bronchitis and is part of chronic obstructive pulmonary disease (COPD). You will cough and produce phlegm most of the time.

Worsen quality of life

- Airways get narrower and this makes it more difficult for air to flow in and out.
- You will have problems breathing and will often feel short of breath,
- The air sacs in your lungs, called alveoli, will gradually be destroyed.
- The oxygen that you breathe in is transferred from the alveoli into your bloodstream, so if alveoli have been destroyed, the lungs are less able to provide the body with oxygen. This is called emphysema.
- Activities where breathing is important will become more and more difficult.
- If you continue to smoke you may even become breathless at rest.

Cause death
- 90% of all deaths from COPD are caused by cigarette smoking.
- 90% of lung cancer deaths in men and almost 80% of lung cancer deaths in women are caused by smoking, as the toxic substances contained in cigarette smoke can cause cells in the airway to become malignant.

- Smoking not only damages your lungs, but also many other vital parts of your body. It causes bad breath, accelerates skin aging, reduces fertility and causes impotence.

Why is nicotine so addictive? Immediate effects

- Sends nicotine to your brain within 10 seconds.
- Makes you feel more calm and alert.
- You enjoy the feeling so you continue to smoke.

Just one puff... Long-term effects

- The chemical structure of your brain changes - it wants more nicotine to have the same effect.
- You become addicted – you associate your daily routine with cravings to make sure you get a steady flow of nicotine.
- The role of cigarettes becomes important in your life as the brain consistently looks for a nicotine fix.

Benefits of Quitting

Levels of toxic substances that are carried to your lungs in cigarette smoke will drop to those of a non-smoker within a few days, which means your lungs will be able to take in more oxygen, which will make it easier for you to breathe.

After a few weeks your airways will become less inflamed, which means you will cough less, produce less phlegm and you will gradually find it easier to exercise.

Long-term damage to your lungs will stop the moment you give up. Severely damaged lungs cannot return to normal, but by quitting before serious damage is done, you can prevent diseases such as COPD getting worse. If you remain cigarette-free you will:

- Reduce your risk of being severely breathless and disabled or dying from COPD.
- Reduce your chance of developing lung cancer. After 15–20 years, the risk of lung cancer is reduced substantially compared with people who continue to smoke.

How can you quit smoking?

Quit Date

No one pretends giving up smoking is easy, but if you have made up your mind to quit you can succeed. It is important to set a date on which you plan to quit smoking (quit-date) and mentally prepare to achieve you set out goal. Use simple tricks to reduce your urge to smoke and help you quit. Look for triggers and plan to avoid them. Consider nicotine replacement therapy or other pharmacotherapeutic agents (Table 5). If you need information or support please call 1-800 QUITNOW.

Here are some other helpful Quit Tips

Do not smoke any number or any kind of cigarettes. Smoking even a few cigarettes a day can hurt your health. If you try to smoke fewer cigarettes but do not stop completely, soon you will be smoking same amount again. Smoking 'low tar, low nicotine' cigarette usually does little good either. As nicotine is so addictive, if you switch to lower nicotine brands you will likely just puff harder, longer and more often on each cigarette. The only safe choice is to quit completely.

Write down why you want to quit. Do you want to feel in control of your life? Be healthier? Set a good example for your children? Protect your family from breathing smoke? Really wanting to quit smoking is very important to how much success you will have in quitting. It is well known that smokers usually quit after a life threatening illness like cancer and heart attack. The reason is that they suddenly become motivated after a health scare. Thus find a reason for quitting before you have no choice.

Know that it will take effort to quit smoking. Nicotine is addictive. Half the battle is knowing that you need to quit and that will help you to deal with the symptoms of withdrawal. You must give yourself a month to get over these feelings. Take quitting one day at a time, one minute at a time.

Don't feel bad if it takes you more than one attempt. There is no "cure" for smoking. It is more like managing a chronic disease. Most people go through cycles of stopping and re-starting the habit, which reflects the strength of your addiction. It is not failure. The good news is that each time you try to quit you are more likely to succeed. Counseling and medication increases your chances. Combining counseling and medication is the most effective. Half of all adult smokers have quit. You can, too, that is the good news. When others can do it, you can succeed too. Get Help if you need. If you need help with nicotine replacement products or other medications please discuss with your physician or dentist.

How to Prevent Relapses of Smoking

- Remind yourself why you gave up smoking in the first place.
- Move away from the area of smokers.
- Keep busy to distract your mind: daily exercise is a good 'distraction' to promote continued abstinence, while counteracting weight gain.
- Drink plenty of water and take deep breaths.

Beware

Some triggers for smoking only reveal themselves after you try to live without cigarettes. Tricks that work for some people may not work for others, so quitting can involve trial and error. Keep going! Ask your doctor or nurse for help. Contact a telephone or internet helpline. The most important thing is to be determined and to persist.

If at first you don't succeed, try again...

Nicotine addiction is very powerful and only 5–10% of 'quit attempts' are successful. Withdrawal symptoms, such as craving, irritability, inability to sleep, mood swings, hunger and headache, that occur when the brain is looking for a new fix of nicotine, are a common reason for relapsing and treatment can help this.

Treatment options

Nicotine replacement products such as gum, patches, inhalers and lozenges can help relieve withdrawal symptoms by delivering small, measured doses of nicotine into your body. Evidence shows that anti-smoking medications can double or even triple your chances of being able to quit. An alternative treatment which doctors recommend for heavy smokers are non-nicotine drugs, such as Buproprion SR (Zyban®) and Varenicline tartrate (Chantix®). They are also effective in relieving the cravings and withdrawal symptoms. The idea of taking a drug to kick a drug habit can make people nervous. Some fear unpleasant side effects, while others fear that one addiction will replace another. But smoking is so dangerous for your health that, if you weigh up the options, (i.e. taking medication or continuing to smoke), using drugs to help you give up smoking will almost always be safer. (See Table 7)

Electronic Cigarettes

Electronic cigarettes or e-cigarettes are electronic nicotine delivery systems (ENDS) that are meant to simulate and substitute for traditional smoking implements, such as cigarettes or cigars, in their use and/or appearance. It generally utilizes a heating element that vaporizes a liquid. Some release nicotine, while others merely release flavored vapor. It substitutes the hand to mouth ritual that most smokers are used to. The risks and benefits of electronic cigarettes are uncertain but they are prescribed as a smoking cessation device.

Table 7: Smoking Cessation Medications

Medications	Dose	Duration	Adverse Effects
Varenicline	1 mg bid	12 weeks if quit attempt, can be extended another 12 weeks.	Nausea
Bupropion SR (slow release)	150 mg every day for 3 d. then 150 mg BID (begin 1-2 weeks pre-quit)	7-12 weeks, maintenance up to 6 months	Insomnia, dry mouth Caution: history of seizures disorder
Nicotine gum	2 or 4 mg gum	Up to 12 weeks	Mouth sores
Nicotine inhaler	6-16 cartridges/day	Up to 6 months	Irritation of mouth & throat
Nicotine nasal spray	8-40 doses/day	3-6 months	Nasal irritation
Nicotine patch	7 -21 mg patch	2-4 weeks	Local skin irritation, insomnia
Nicotine Lozenges	2 -4 mg lozenge	8 weeks	Mouth sores

Chapter 11

Diet and Nutrition

"No disease that can be treated by diet should be treated with any other means."

Maimonides (1135-1204)

Proper nutrition contributes to overall wellness and is essential for individuals with chronic lung disease. A healthy body is better able to fight off infections, thus preventing simple colds from progressing into a more serious lung infection. If illness does occur, a well-nourished body helps to produce a better response to treatment and therefore help you get better faster. You may consult a nutritionist, especially if you are dealing with additional problems such as heart disease or diabetes. The discussion

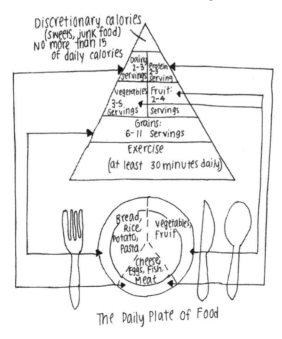

The Healthy Eating Pyramid

The Daily Plate of Food

in this chapter is general but please consult your physician for your individual needs

Nutrition and Lung Disease

A healthy person should aim to get 45% to 65% of their calories from carbohydrates, with active individuals aiming for 55% to 65%. As for protein a healthy individual should aim to get about 10% to 35% of their calories. Fats are also essential to our well being, a healthy individual should aim to get 20% to 35% of their calories from fat.

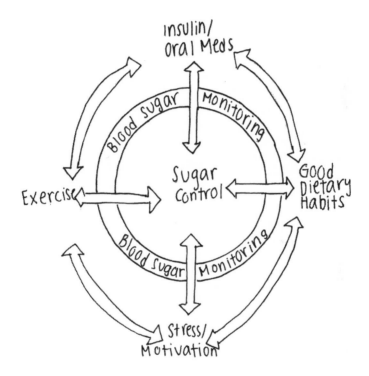

Proteins

While protein can be used for energy when carbohydrates and fat are in short supply, protein's major role is building muscle, make blood and other body tissues. Many people consume meat products as a source of protein. It is important to know red meats such as beef are linked to increased risk of heart disease. Good sources of protein include eggs, poultry (white meat), soy and whey.

Carbohydrates

Carbohydrates are the body's main source of energy. They may come in the form of simple sugars such as sucrose and fructose or in wheat products such as breads and pastas. Eating extra carbohydrate gives runners energy, but it will give patients with history of lung disease carbon dioxide.

Fats

Fats are a common component of many foods. It is important to keep in mind that not all fats are bad and they might not be associated with cholesterol. Foods that are high in cholesterol and saturated fats come mostly from animal sources. To differentiate between saturated and unsaturated fats you can see how they act at certain temperatures. Saturated fats turn solid in cool temperatures for example butter or the layer of fat on top of a pot of chicken soup that's been in the refrigerator. Polyunsaturated fats do not contain cholesterol. These are fats are from plant sources and they remain liquid at cold temperatures for example olive oil.

When you consume fat, make an effort that it is the polyunsaturated kind. Avoid animal fats such as butter and cut down on fatty meats, as these foods are high in cholesterol. Before you buy prepared products, read the labels. Many prepared foods list the cholesterol content on the ingredient panel. If you can buy either a product made with butter or one made with corn oil, choose the one made with corn oil.

More recently as a community we have become of aware of a different type of fat called a trans fats. Trans fats are a type of unsaturated fat that have a different chemical configuration than typical saturated and unsaturated fats. These trans fats are created by the processing and hydrogenation of unsaturated fats. These types of fats may be found naturally in the plant kingdom and in certain meat products like beef. Trans fats have been associated with increased incidence of cardiac disease. They should be avoided whenever possible.

Table 8: Healthy vs. Less Healthy Fats

Healthy Fats	Less Healthy or Unhealthy Fats
Monounsaturated Fats • Olive oil • Peanut oil • Sesame oil • Variety of nut and seed oils: peanut, almond, macadamia nut, sesame • Avocados, olives • Full-fat ice cream	**Saturated Fats** • Butter • Lard • Tropical oils such as coconut, palm, palm kernel, cocoa butter • Fatty meats • Whole milk
Polyunsaturated Fats • Corn oil • Soybean oil • Sunflower oil • Safflower oil • Oil found in fish, salmon, tuna, mackerel, sardines, herring, anchovies • Variety of nut and seed oils: walnut, pumpkin, flax • Heart-healthy spreads, such as Benecol and Take Control (if used two to three times a day in place of regular margarine or butter, these products may lower cholesterol by up to 14 percent	**Trans (Hydrogenated) Fats** • Shortening • Hard stick margarine (check labels) • Many baked goods, especially processed ones (check labels): croissants, doughnuts, muffins, biscuits, chips, crackers, cookies, cakes • Many fried foods, such as French fries, chicken nuggets, fish sticks

Portion Control

Portion control is an important part of any diet and weight management plan. Our stomachs have adapted to our diet and lifestyle over many years. When you eat a really large meal the diaphragm cannot move as far down, so the lungs do not fill as well. Instead of eating three big meals a day, try dividing your day's food into five or six smaller portions. This way, your stomach will not fill as much after each meal. You can eat a smaller breakfast, lunch and dinner and supply the rest of your nutritional needs for the day by having two or three small snacks.

Ideal Body Weight

It is possible to eat your way to a great health. General guidelines you need to follow are: getting rid of junk food, consuming sufficient protein (the USDA recommends 10-30 grams a day). The protein in diet and it should be from poultry or plant based protein saturated fat, high sodium food, prepackaged food

Weight loss is a common problem in patients with advanced lung disease. One reason is that more calories than normal are used for routine breathing. A person with lung disease can burn 10 times as many calories just breathing as does a healthy person. Following the above mentioned suggestions it is important to try to achieve an ideal body weight.

Shed Excess Weight

In the setting of advanced lung disease it is important to shed excess weight. The work of breathing in increased in certain conditions like COPD and pulmonary hypertension and not as efficient in conditions like interstitial lung disease. Any additional weight may make your breathing worse. Increased mass not only increases the stress on your lungs but also your heart. Extra body weight demands more oxygen and can interfere with breathing.

Get in the habit of weighing yourself regularly. Not only will the scale tell you if you're getting heavier, it will also alert you that you may not be eating enough. You should see your doctor or dietitian if you continue to lose weight while following the recommended diet. It is also recommended to join a medical weight loss group. When weight loss is considered is it important to keep in mind that a BMI of 25 is preferred.

You should also maintain a 1200-1700 diet and make sure that you are following with a nutritionist.

Gaining weight in Advanced Lung Disease

Sometimes in advanced lung disease it is difficult to maintain an ideal body weight. The lack of oxygenation will cause you body to lose muscle mass. Your nutritionist or doctor may suggest you drink a liquid meal supplement. Many people with high nutritional needs add a medical nutritional product to their diet. These products are so nutritious that they can be used as a complete diet by people who are unable to eat normal foods, or they can be added to regular foods for people who cannot eat enough.

Salt and Fluid Intake

United Stated Drug Administration (USDA) guidelines include recommendations for the general population. It has been recommended that no one should consume more than 2,300 milligrams of salt per day. Those who are age 51 and older and those who are African American or have high blood pressure, diabetes or chronic kidney disease should consume no more than 1,500 milligrams per day.

As for fluid intake the amount of fluid in your body is related to your consumption of fluid and particularly to your sodium intake. Sodium intake can greatly affect your fluid retention and may increase blood pressure and exacerbate heart and lung disease. Remember that some foods are full of liquid. For example, a cup of gelatin dessert has almost as much water as a cup of juice.

Hints to Reduce Salt/Sodium

Excessive salt/sodium intake may cause your body to retain fluid. This extra fluid volume often increases blood volume. It then becomes more difficult for your heart to circulate the blood. Breathing may become more difficult to keep up with the extra energy needs.

- Take the salt shaker off the table, only use during cooking.
- Flavor with herbs and spices, onions, garlic and pepper.

- Use fresh meats, fruits and vegetables. Processed foods are usually high in sodium.
- Read food labels and avoid products which use the words salt, sodium, Na or soda in the first three ingredients.
- Consult your physician before using salt substitutes.

Rest just before eating

The time you rest has a great impact on when you should eat. Eat your main meal early if you are usually too tired to eat later in the day. Avoid foods that cause gas or bloating. They will make your breathing more difficult. Your dietitian or doctor may suggest that you replace some of the carbohydrate in your diet with fat, since less carbon dioxide results from eating fat than from eating carbohydrates. Foods such as sugar, candy, jelly, jam and sugar-containing desserts contain a lot of carbohydrate but little protein and few vitamins and minerals. By replacing some of these foods with others a dietitian suggests, you are reducing carbohydrate that you don't need. Other foods such as breads, vegetables and fruits also contain carbohydrates, but they have other important nutrients, so you will want to continue eating them. You can avoid some unnecessary carbohydrates in these foods. For example, by using fresh fruit or canned fruit packed in juice or water rather than in heavy syrup.

Here are some other suggestions to help you limit the amount of carbohydrate and increase your intake of good fats

- Eat enough calories to attain and maintain desired body weight.
- Eat fewer foods high in fat. These include: dairy and meat products, fried foods, oils, sauces, salad dressings, granola, party crackers and dips, fast foods, convenience foods and commercial pastries.
- Use artificial sweeteners.
- Eat a balanced diet and a variety of foods at each meal. "Balanced" means a protein source (meat or dairy product, beans or peas), carbohydrates (fruits, vegetables, grains and starches), fats (oil or margarine) and fluid at each meal.
- Substitute polyunsaturated fats for saturated fats whenever possible. Saturated fats are usually animal fats, found in dairy and meat products (such as butter, cream cheese, creamy salad

dressings, visible and "hidden" meat fat, bacon, luncheon meats, sausage and hot dogs, fried foods), but sometimes are vegetable fats, as in chocolate, or coconut and palm oils. Polyunsaturated fats are only from vegetable sources: vegetable oils and margarine (especially tub margarines), nuts, avocados, olives and unhydrogenated peanut butter. Eat more fish, poultry and veal in place of beef, lamb, pork and cheese. Use sunflower, corn, sunflower, soybean and cottonseed oils and margarines.

- Eat more complex carbohydrates and less refined, simple sugars. Complex carbohydrates are: fresh fruits and vegetables, whole-grained and enriched cereals (bread, cereals, rice, pasta, grits, oatmeal, cracked wheat and bran), potatoes, corn, peas, beans, lentils. Simple sugars are: sugar, honey, jam, jelly, sodas, candy, cookies, cake, processed foods and beverages, sugar-coated cereals. Eat complex carbohydrates for vitamins, minerals, energy, fiber, water and fewer calories.
- Use water-packed fruit or fruit with no added sugar.
- Use artificially sweetened jams, jellies and hard candies.
- If you have certain favorite foods you are not sure about, ask your dietitian if they are high in carbohydrate. Your dietitian may suggest ways that other foods can be used to balance the carbohydrate in those things you most enjoy.

Fiber

Fiber is a portion of vegetables, fruits, grains and beans which passes through our digestive tract into the large intestine nearly completely undigested. Fiber aids bowel function, weight control and may play a role in reducing cholesterol levels and carbohydrates absorption. Foods that are high in fiber include:

- Whole grain breads and cereals: bran, whole wheat, rye and pumpernickel
- Fresh fruits, fresh vegetables and salads
- Legumes: chick peas, lentils, beans, peas, etc.

Beverages

Drinking 6-8 glasses of fluid a day helps to keep mucous thin and easier to cough up. Water, low calorie fruit juices, decaffeinated coffee or tea and milk are recommended beverages. Milk does not cause thickened saliva as many believe. Alcohol, fruit-flavored drinks and soft drinks should be avoided since they are high in calories and contain little nutritional value.

Vitamin Supplements

Vitamin supplements are not necessary if you follow a well balanced diet. If you habitually eat a poor balanced diet you may benefit from a multi-vitamin. Consult your physician prior to beginning a new vitamin regimen.

Changing Your Habits

A lot of your health maintenance is up to you. As you have you read the previous chapters you know that changing some habits to take better care of yourself may help your lung disease. Maybe you'd like to change some of your habits but you're stuck and you feel as if it is very hard to start. Changing habits can be hard to do. But you can learn a step-by-step approach that will help you reach your goals.

How can you start to change your habits?

Every change involved several stages:

- Precontemplation - Maybe you think that a change would help but you're not ready or interested. You feel the change would be too hard to make.
- Contemplation - You're thinking about making a change, but not right away. At this stage, the costs of making the change still outweigh the benefits.
- Preparation - You're ready to make the change within the month. You've made a realistic plan and you've gathered what you need to carry out your plan.
- Action - You've taken action and started your new routine. But sometimes you're tempted to go back to your previous habits.
- Maintenance - After more than 6 months of your new routine, you're used to doing it. It's now a habit.

To change a habit, you have to realize what stage you are in. Once you have established which stage you are you can better

Diet and Weight Management Pearls

- To limit the amount of food you consume in a sitting drink a full glass of water (8 ounces) immediately prior to eating. This water will take up some space in the stomach and stretch it triggering fullness centers in the brain. This will trick your mind into thinking that you do not need much more food to be full.
- Drink six to eight glasses of water a day. Proper hydration allows your body to shed any excess water that is stored in your fat cells. Not only will you lose your water weight but you body will function more efficiently.
- Start eating your meals out of smaller vessels. For example instead of having dinner in a full sized dinner plate start using a quarter plate. The purpose of this is to trick your mind into thinking that you have already had a sufficient portion. When going back for a second serving your mind will alert you that you are getting a second serving.
- Pre-cut vegetables into snack size portions. Place them in Ziploc sandwich back and keep them in the refrigerator front and center. This technique allows you to quickly open the fridge and get a snack that is healthy and delicious without much thinking. It also prevents you from eating some unhealthy snack like ice cream or chips and dip.
- Label the calories on all food with a big bold marker. Labeling all the items in your fridge with the calories will let you see how many calories you will get from a particular for before you grab it. The same goes for all pantry items and prepared foods.

What is a Serving?

While planning on how to count your calories and manage your portion sizes it is important to have an idea of what exactly a serving is. Most food items have nutritional information on them that is based on a serving. A serving may be different for different foods. Below find a table that tries to simplify what is a serving.

Everyday household items can be used as guidelines for healthy serving sizes!

Household Item	Serving	Food
Deck of Cards	3-4 Ounces	Beef, Chicken, Pork, Salmon
Checkbook	~3 Ounces	Lean Fish Fillet
Compact Disk	~1 Ounce	Lunchmeat Pancake Waffle
Baseball	1 Cup	Cooked Pasta Cold Cereal Raw Vegetable
Tennis Ball	½ Cup	Cooked Vegetable Ice Cream Piece of Fruit

Golf Ball 	~2 Tablespoons ~1/4 Cup	Peanut Butter Dried fruit, nuts
4 Dice 	~1 Ounce	Cheese
Computer Mouse 	1 Small	Potato
Your thumb 	1 Tablespoon	Olive Oil Dressing Mayonnaise

Chapter 12

Traveling with Lung Disease

"Nobody travels on the road to success without a puncture or two."

Navjot Singh Sidhu (b. 1963)

As with any other aspect of living with advanced lung disease, planning ahead and taking precaution can allow you to travel with a free mind. It's good to get out of the house and enjoy life.

What precautions should I take when traveling?

- When you travel alone make sure you travel light and have the appropriate luggage.
- When you travel make sure you plan your route in advance. You should plan a route that reduces your lung and oxygen expenditure.
- Make you sure you keep your cell phone with you at ALL times. This may your only lifeline to call for help if need be.
- Travel at times when traffic is light to cut down travel time.
- On long trips every hour you should exercise your legs to prevent blood clots from forming.
- Stay hydrated by drinking non-alcoholic, non-caffeinated beverages.
- When making hotel reservations or other accommodation, make sure your needs are met (elevators, ramps, etc.)
- Before traveling to a particular city make a list of clinics, hospitals and health centers that will be close to where you are staying.
- If possible, book direct flights. This allows you to avoid any layovers where oxygen may not be available.
- Have your immunizations up to date. In addition keep an extra supply of your medications. Bring enough medication to cover your needs in case of a long delay or lost bags.

- Check your health insurance coverage and travel insurance policy to make sure that any medical costs that may arise will be covered.
- It can be a long, tiring walk to the departure gate, but you can ask for wheelchair or electric cart. Notify the airline when you make your airline reservation and confirm your request on the departure day. Before you board the plane, you will be using your own portable oxygen unit. You may need a family member or your oxygen supplier to pick up your portable oxygen unit that you will leave at the gate.
- Keep a current list of your medications while traveling.
- Bring the phone numbers of your health care providers, including your physician, respiratory therapist and oxygen supplier.
- Always travel with your complete identification including medical information (medical alert bracelet, device identification card, etc)

What about Air Travel?

Air travel is something that has become commonplace, even with patients with advanced medical conditions. Some patients with advanced lung disease may require additional evaluation prior to air travel. Anyone whose lung disease is serious enough to warrant oxygen use may have to undergo further lung testing to assess readiness for flight. The gold standard test to evaluate readiness for flight is called the Hypoxia-Altitude Simulation Test (HAST). This test will see if you're able to be at reduced atmospheric pressures associated with high altitude air travel.

During air travel cabin pressure can affect the health and well-being of passengers in many ways, including hypobaric hypoxia affecting those with pre-existing respiratory conditions such as heart failure. It may also cause gas expansion within body cavities and medical devices. Although commercial flights usually cruise at altitudes of 5000 m above sea level, the passenger cabin is pressurized to an altitude of 1500-2500 m. Most regulatory governmental agencies require the cabin altitude not to exceed 2400 m.

Your doctor can determine if you will need oxygen during your flight by attaching an oximeter to your finger which measures how much oxygen you have in your blood. If the oxygen in your blood is low, there's a danger that your oxygen will drop further and to prevent this from happening, you must have supplemental oxygen available on your flight. Since 2005, portable oxygen concentrators, which concentrate oxygen in ambient air by removing nitrogen content, have become available as an alternative to traditional oxygen cylinders. Passengers need a signed doctor's statement of medical necessity and notify the airline before travelling. For a list of approved devices please refer to the Federal Aviation Administration website or ask your physician. In the United States, since 2008 due to modification of the US Government Air Carrier Access Act in May all US-based air carriers and foreign air carrier flights that begin or end in the can accommodate passengers who need portable oxygen concentrators.

Chapter 13

Lung Disease and Social Life

"The biggest disease this day and age is that of people feeling unloved."

Princess Diana (1961-1997)

A diagnosis of chronic lung disease may cause you to feel sad and worried about your future. These feelings may manifest as depression, which may have a detrimental effect on your overall health. Depression is a condition that is caused by a combination of psychological, physical and in some case genetic factors. In lung disease physical limitations play a major role in the precipitation of negative thoughts which are a precursor to development of depression

Patients with both lung disease and depression are more likely to be hospitalized for lung-related symptoms. Depression can also make it difficult to take care of yourself and your disease properly. When this feeling sets in, you may also want to stop fighting your disease and miss medications. You may think that it is pointless to exercise, or that they are not able to do enough to make a difference. All this can make lung disease worse.

Depression

The symptoms of depression are commonly described by the acronym SIG-E-CAPS. You must have 2 or more of the following symptoms on most days for at least 2 weeks duration to have a diagnose of depression

- Sleep changes: increase during day or decreased sleep at night
- Interest (loss): of interest in activities that used to interest them
- Guilt (worthless): depressed elderly tend to devalue themselves
- Energy (lack): common presenting symptom (fatigue)
- Cognition/Concentration: reduced cognition &/or difficulty concentrating

- Appetite (wt. loss); usually declined, occasionally increased
- Psychomotor: agitation (anxiety) or retardations (lethargic)
- Suicidal thoughts

Management of Depression

Depression may be managed in many ways. The first step to management is acknowledging the way you feel and actively seeking help. Conservatively it may be managed by talking to someone. This may be a family member, a psychologist or you may even attend a support group meeting. Depression may also be managed with cognitive behavior therapy (CBT), a form of psychotherapy that trains people to view their feelings in a more positive way and to cope with the stresses of living with a chronic disease. Some people may fine the above therapies enough but others may also need to use anti-depressant medications (See Appendix 5). Antidepressant medications work by changing the concentration of neurotransmitters (signaling chemicals) in the brain. These medications take some time to reach their effective levels and may take up to one month before you see results. Eventually these medications may be able to restore your sense of well-being. More recently is has been shown that physical activity improves mental well-being. Living with advanced lung disease, physical activity may benefit both your mental and physical health.

In addition sex is an important part of social life, marriage and relationships. Advance lung disease can disturb this whole aspect of a relationship and can be caused on either or both partners feel there is trouble. Discuss this with each other, is important as it can keep each other informed about your feelings. Remember having advanced lung disease doesn't mean that sexual activity must be reduced, curtailed or totally eliminated.

Chapter 14

Problems of Caregiving

"Caregiving has no second agendas or hidden motives. The care is given from love for the joy of giving without expectation, no strings attached."

Gary Zukav (b. 1942)

Caregivers of patients with advanced lung disease are people who take care, most often parents or spouses, who are ill or disabled. Often they participate in both direct (physician appointments, medications, etc.) and indirect patient care (groceries, cooking, etc.) It is estimated that approximately 60 million Americans are caregivers to some capacity. The National Family Caregiving Association found that 61% of caregivers providing at least 20 hours of caregiving per week suffered from depression.

Depression in caregivers is due to the intertwined nature of medical, social and economic factors. Often caregivers, taking care of loved ones become over consumed with their responsibilities and forget to take care of their mental and physical well-being. The difficult nature of taking care of advanced lung disease patients and their behaviors such as anger and aggressiveness may increase the incidence of caregiver depression more so than cognitive impairment.

Caregivers can seek outside help from home health aides, especially in physically demanding care situations or negotiating with other family members and friends to take over while the primary caregiver takes regular breaks to get relief. Joining support groups and checking to see whether the local hospital offers supplemental home health care, caregiver training, or other services can help.

Not everyone reacts to the responsibility of being a caregiver equally. People who care for their spouses are more prone to caregiving-related stress than those who care for other family members.

Signs and Symptoms of Caregivers Stress

- Change in Sleeping habits - sleeping too much or too little.
- Change in eating habits - resulting in weight gain or loss.
- Feeling of apathy, tiredness and fatigue.
- Loss of interest in activities you normally enjoy.
- You get easily irritated, angered, or saddened

Get the Help You Need: Find out about community caregiving resources (transportation services, visiting nurse services). You may also look for faith-based groups for help and support. Transportation services may also be available to you.

Communicate Clearly: Stay in touch with friends and family. In addition social activities can help you feel connected and may reduce stress.

Take Scheduled Breaks: Find time for exercise and try to get enough sleep. It is important to also take one day at a time.

Take Care of Yourself and Accept Help: It is important not to forget to Prioritize, make lists and establish a daily routine. Make sure to see your doctor for routine checkups and talk about symptoms of depression or sickness you may be having. Don't forget to exercise regularly and live a healthy lifestyle. Be ready to accept help from family, medical professionals and the community.

What is respite care?

Respite care refers to the mental well-being and attention that caregiver needs. Caregivers may look for outlets or temporary assistance in various ways while they take a "breather" from care of a loved one. Some optional assistance programs for direct patient care are: Home health care services (Visiting Nurse Services), Adult day-care centers (Senior Centers), Assisted living homes and Support groups

Similarly caregivers may reach out into the community for assistance involving transportation, meals, adult day care, home care, cleaning and yard work services, home modification, senior centers, hospice care, support groups, legal and financial counseling.

Chapter 15

Managing Lung Disease at Home

"We are not victims of aging, sickness and death. These are part of scenery, not the seer, who is immune to any form of change. This seer is the spirit, the expression of eternal being."

Deepak Chopra (b. 1947)

To help manage your disease you should first talk to your family members about what you need to do to have a good day. Begin by reviewing the following information. Together, talk to the doctor or nurse about keeping an adequate supply of prescription medications on hand.

Always be prepared:
- You should always have adequate supply of routine medications. In addition, set aside medications to treat shortness of breath, pain and sudden cough.
- Identify a health care agent (family member or friend) or a proxy to help make emergent medical decisions.
- Complete an advanced directive form in case you do not want to be intubated and/or resuscitative measures performed in emergent situations
- Adequate oxygen supply (cylinders, concentrators, supplies, etc.), if ordered by the physician
- Make sure your durable medical devices (CPAP machine, nebulizer machine, inhalation devices) are always in working order.
- All important medical and family phone numbers should be on the refrigerator and easy to find.

Tips for Coping with Acute Episodes of Dyspnea

- Assess severity of the episode by rating how short of breath you feel on a scale of 1 to 10.
- Monitor changes in your body that alerts you to increased shortness of breath. Call health care provider if shortness of breath changes in frequency and intensity. If you have asthma, measure peak flow rate with a peak flow meter. If the value is lower than your baseline, use a metered dose inhaler with sustained inspiration and breath holding. Take a second puff of medication and then measure peak flow rate gain. Tell your health care provider the values you have recorded when you call.
- Use all the techniques you have learned to decrease your shortness of breath such as pursed-lip breathing, relaxation, abdominal breathing, position, fluids, fans and medications, including those delivered by nebulizers. Simple relaxation or meditation strategies may help you relax and permit slower, deeper breathing, thus allowing a sense of control over breathing.
- Evaluate your response to the strategies and medications you have tried. If symptoms have not markedly improved, proceed to the doctor's office, clinic, or emergency room without delay.
- Make duplicates of all keys. Bury a house key in a secret spot in the garden or carry a duplicate car key in your wallet, apart from your key ring.
- Practice preventive maintenance. Your car, appliances, home and relationships will be less likely to break down/fall apart "at the worst possible moment."
- Procrastination is stressful. Whatever you want to do tomorrow, do today, whatever you want to do today, do it now.
- Allow 15 minutes of extra time to get to appointments. Plan to arrive at an airport two hours before domestic departures.
- Ask questions. Taking a few moments to repeat back directions, what someone expects of you, etc. can save hours.

Don't Panic

Shortness of breath or other symptoms can be frightening. Keep calm and try to calm your loved one. Remember, help is just a phone call away. Call your physician's office or 911!

By keeping track of basic information, you will be able to provide the doctor with accurate and up-to-date reports, either over the phone or during visits. This record does not need to be complicated. In fact, the simpler, the better. A spiral-bound notebook or composition book will do just fine. Have your loved one get in the habit of routinely recording the following information:

- Precipitating factors of shortness of breath (walking, stair climbing, anxiety, upper respiratory infections, etc.)
- List of medications-names, doses, list of all allergies.
- Other symptoms to discuss with your doctor, such as daily weight and leg swelling.
- Swollen hands, ankles, or feet
- Increased fatigue, chest pain, fainting spells, sleep disruption
- Shortness of breath that interrupts sleep

Chapter 16

<u>End of Life Issues</u>

"Faith consists in believing when it is beyond the power of reason to believe."

Voltaire (1694 – 1778)

What is an Advance Directive?

An advance directive (i.e. Health Care Proxy Card) is a legal document in which you specify what type of medical care you want in the future, or whom you want to make healthcare decisions for you, if you become medically unable to do so. Advance directive allows you to maintain control over your own medical care at a time you can't communicate yourself.

What is a Health Care Agent?

A health care agent (also called a proxy) is someone you appoint to make healthcare decisions for you when you are medically unable to. If you choose to name a health care agent, he or she can decide how your wishes apply as your medical condition changes. You may give the person you select as your health care agent as little or as much authority as you want by explaining your wishes in your advance directive. Be sure that your health care agent knows what is important to you. A health care agent can agree to treatment, choose between different treatments and/or refuse or withdraw treatment.

Appointment a health care agent lets you control your medical treatment by:

- Allowing your agent to make healthcare decisions on your behalf as you would want them decided;
- Choosing one person to make healthcare decisions because you think that person would make the best decisions based on your beliefs and medical circumstances;

- Avoiding conflict or confusion among family members and/or significant others.

Who needs an Advance Directive?

Having an advance directive and appointing a health care agent is a good idea for everyone over the age of 18. Being too ill or confused to make medical decisions can happen at any age. A health care agent can act on your behalf if you become temporarily unable to make your own health care decisions (such as might occur if you are under general anesthesia or have become comatose because of an accident). In New York State, only the health care agent you appoint has the legal authority to make treatment decisions if you are unable to for yourself.

Who can be a Health Care Agent?

Anyone 18 years of age or older can be a health care agent. The individual can be a spouse/significant other, family member, friend or someone else you trust to make health care decisions on your behalf.

How do you complete an Advance Directive?

Ask your health care provider for a New York State Health Care Proxy Form. If you want to expand on any specific wishes or preferences or want to limit authority in any way, please see your health care provider for the larger New York State Health Care Proxy Form. Give a copy of the Health Care Proxy form to your health care agent, your physicians, your attorney and any other family members or close friends.

What if you change your mind?

If you decide to cancel your Health Care Proxy Card, to change the person you have chosen as your agent or to alter any instructions or limitations you have included on the car, simple destroy the card, complete a new one and notify all those who have copies.

Medical Orders for Life-Sustaining Treatment (MOLST) form

Honoring patients' preferences is a critical step in providing quality end of life care. Physicians and other health care providers, use the MOLST form on the belief that as a patient you have the right to determine what treatments you want to receive in serious and end of life situations. It is a bright pink form that allows physicians and health care providers, including emergency medical services (EMS), to follow your wishes regarding receiving cardio-pulmonary resuscitation (CPR) or any other life sustaining treatment. MOLST is intended for patients with serious conditions, who don't want any life sustaining treatments, stay in a long term facility such nursing homes or may die within a year. The first step in completing this form is talking with your family or health care proxy along with a qualified trained health care professional who will explain the details about completing this form as well as treatment options. If you move from one state to another, all health care professionals must follow these orders. You should talk to your health care provider and/or visit government websites to get more information about the MOLST form

Grief

Grief is something we must all experience at some point in our lives but it helps to know the feeling and how others have coped with it. The grief process occurs many times during the course of an illness, both before and after the death of someone you love. Here are a few suggestions on how to live through grief, ways to grieve with and for the dying person and how to cope during difficult times, such as holidays, birthdays and other anniversary dates. Throughout the course of a life-ending illness, you will encounter many milestones and with each, experience some degree of loss. With loss, in general, comes grief and sadness. Below are a few notes that helped people cope with their feelings of grief.

Solitude helps. You may need time to think about your loved one, to remember times you shared, to consider how your life will be now. You may be overwhelmed by your sorrow. You may want to stay in bed and cry or sleep, go for a walk, or sit in a chapel.

Seek Family and Friends. These people are likely to empathize with you. Even if they do not know what to say, just being with other people and talking can be supportive. Accept others' invitations to participate in activities, but leave if you feel you need to. Reach out to family or friends when the next hour or day seems unbearable.

Meditation helps. In a time of emotional and mental distress clearing your thoughts may help with the grief process. Activities like meditation and prayer may make the grief process more bearable.

Rest and sleep help. Caring for a dying person is exhausting. You may need time alone simply to regain your physical energy, as well as your emotional and spiritual strength. Routines help. Even though your life may feel turned upside down, try to keep up a routine of healthy eating, occasional physical activity (even a 10-minute walk) and regular sleep.

Time helps. Your life may never be the same again. Whatever your experience with death and dying, you will find that you see the world and your place in it differently. Time lessens some of grief's pain, but it does not diminish your loss or sadness

Appendix

Appendix 1: List of Antibiotics

Antibiotics	Generic	Brand Name ®
Penicillins	Penicillin V, G	
	Amoxicillin	
	Ampicillin	
	Amoxicilln/Clavuanate	Augmentin
	Ampicillin/Sulbactam	Unasyn
Penicillin Resistant	Nafcillin	
	Oxacillin	
	Dicloxacillin	
Anti-Pseudomonal	Peperacillin/Tazobactam	Zosyn
	Ticarcillin/Clavulanate	Timentin
Carbepenams	Imepenem/Cilastatin	Primaxin
	Meropenem	Merrem
	Ertapenem	Invanz
Monobactams	Aztreonam	Azactam
Cephalosporins		
1st Generation	Cefazolin	Ancef
	Cehalexin	Keflex
	Cefadroxil	Duricef
2nd Generation	Cefotetan	Cefotan
	Cefoxitin	Mefoxin
	Cefuroxime	Ceftin
	Cefprozil	Cefzil
3rd Generation	Cefotaxime	Claforan
	Ceftriaxone	Rocephin
	Ceftazidime	Fortaz
4th Generation	Cefepime	Maxipime
Fluroquinolones	Ciprofloxacin	Cipro
	Levofloxacin	Levaquin
	Moxifloxacin	Avelox
Aminoglycosides	Gentamycin	
	Tobramycin	
	Amikacin	
Microlides	Azithromycin	Zithromax
	Clarithromycin	Biaxin
	Erythromycin	
Tetracyclines	Tetracycline	
	Minocycline	Minocin
	Doxycycline	Vibramycin

Appendix 2: List of Medications Used for Asthma and COPD

Bronchodilator Type	Generic Names	Trade Names®
Bronchodilator Nebulizer	Albuterol	Ventolin, Proventil
	Arformoterol	Brovana
	Levalbuterol	Xopenex
Bronchodilator HFA	Albuterol	Ventolin HFA, Proventil HFA, ProAir HFA
	Levalbuterol	Xopenex HFA
	Pirbutrol	Maxair
Bronchodilator(Anticholiner gics)	Ipratropium Bromide Neb/HFA	Atrovent Neb/HFA
	Tiotropium bromide	Spiriva*
Bronchodilator (Anticholinergic + Beta Agonist)	Ipratropium Bromide with Albuterol	Combivent HFA*
Muscarinic Antagonists	Aclidinium bromide	Tudorza
Corticosteroids	Methylprednisolone	Medrol
	Prednisolone	Orapred
Inhaled Corticosteroids	Beclomethasone HFA	QVar
	Budesonide Neb/DPI	Pulmicort Neb/DPI
	Ciclesonide HFA	Alvesco
	Flunisolide HFA	Aerospan
	Fluticasone DPI/HFA	Flovent DPI/HFA
	Mometasone	Asmanex
Combination Meds (Beta Agonist + Steroids)	Fluticasone/Salmeterol DPI/HFA	Advair DPI/HFA
	Mometasone/Formoter ol HFA	Dulera HFA
	Budesonide/Formoterol HFA	Symbicort HFA
Long Acting Beta 2 Bronchodilators	Salmeterol DPI	Serevent Diskus
	Formoterol DPI	Foradil

Appendix 2: continued

Phosphodiesterase 4 (PDE-4) Inhibitor	Roflumilast	Daliresp
Mast Cell Stabilizers	Cromolyn Sodium	Intal
Leukotriene Receptor Antagonist (LTRAs)	Montelukast	Singulair
	Zafirlukast	Accolate
	Zileuton	Zyflo
Monoclonal Antibody	Olamizumab	Xolair

HFA – Hydrofluoroalkane, DPI – Dry Powdered Inhaler, * Also available with Respimat soft mist inhaler (SMI)

Appendix 3: Recommended Adult Vaccinations

http://www.cdc.gov

Vaccine	Age 18-60	Age 60+
Influenza	One dose annually	One dose annually
Varicella	2 doses	
Zoster		1 dose
Pneumococcal poly saccharine (PPSV23)	1 or 2 doses	1 dose (65+)
Pneumococcal 13-valent conjugate (PCV13)	1 dose	
Measles, Mumps, rubella (MMR)	1 or 2 doses	
Meningococcal	1 or more doses	
Hepatitis A	2 doses	
Hepatitis B	3 doses	

Appendix 4: List of Oral Diabetes Medications

Type of Medicine	Route	How They Work	Dosing Schedule
Meglitinides	Oral	Help beta cells release insulin	1-4 times daily
Sulfonylureas	Oral	Help beta cells release insulin	1 or 2 times daily
Biguanides	Oral	Lower sugar production by the liver	1 or 2 times daily
Thiazolidinediones	Oral	Help Cells and tissues use insulin	1 or 2 times daily
Alpha-Glucosidase Inhibitors	Oral	Slow digestion of sugar	Before each meal
GLP-1 agonists	Injectable	Help beta cells release insulin, stop release of un-needed sugar by liver, slow emptying of the stomach	Inject once or twice daily
DPP-4 Inhibitors	Oral	Help beta cells release insulin and decrease glucagon secretion	Once daily

Appendix 4a: List of Insulin Regimen for Diabetes

Insulin Type	When it's usually taken	How soon it starts working	Peak Effect	Duration
Analog Insulin				
Fast Acting	Right before meal	15 min.	30-90 min.	3-5 hr.
Long Acting	30 min. before evening meal or breakfast	1 hr.	Steady over time	Up to 24 hours
Premixed (mix of fast and intermediate acting)	Before breakfast and/or evening meal	5-15 min.	Varies	Up to 24 hours

Human Insulin				
Short Acting	30 min. before meal	30-60 min.	2-4 hr.	5-8 hours
Intermediate Acting (NPH)	30 min before breakfast and/or evening meal	1-3 hr.	8 hours	Up to 24 hours
Premixed (mixture of short (regular) and NPH insulin	30 min before breakfast and/or evening meal	30-60 min.	Varies	Up to 24 hours

Appendix 5: List of Depression Medications

Type of Medication	Generic Names	Trade Names®
Selective serotonin-reuptake inhibitor *(SSRIs)*	Fluoxetine Sertraline Paroxetine Citalopram Escitalopram Fluvoxamine	Prozac Zoloft Paxil Celexa Lexapro Luvox
Serotonin-norepinephrine reuptake inhibitor *(SNRIs)*	Venlafaxine Duloxetine Desvenlafaxine	Effexor Cymbalta Pristiq
Atypical antidepressant	Bupropion Mirtazepine Trazodone	Wellbutrin, Zyban Remeron Desyrel
Tricyclic antidepressant *(TCAs)*	Amitriptyline Clomipramine Desipramine Doxepine Imipramine Nortriptyline Protriptyline Maprotilin	Elavil Anafranil Norpramin, Sinequan, Adapin Tofranil Aventyl, Pamelor Vivactil, Triptil Ludiomil
Monoamine oxidase inhibitors *(MAOs)*	Isocarboxazid Phenelzine Tranylcypromine	Marplan Nardil Parnate

Useful Contact Information

American College of Chest Physicians
3300 Dundee Road
Northbrook, IL 60062-2348   (847)-498-1400
http://www.chestnet.org/

American Diabetes Association
1701 North Beauregard Street
Alexandria, VA 22311   1-800 DIABETES
http://www.diabetes.org

American Sleep Apnea Association
6856 Eastern Avenue NW Suite 203
Washington, DC 20012   1-888 293-3650
http://www.sleepapnea.org/

American Thoracic Society
25 Broadway, 18th Floor
New York, NY 10004   (212)-315-8600
http://www.thoracic.org/

Coalition for Pulmonary Fibrosis
10866 W. Washington Blvd #343
Culver City, CA 90232   1-888 222-8541
http://www.coalitionforpf.org/

Pulmonary Hypertension Association
801 Roeder Road, Ste. 1000
Silver Spring, MD 20910   (301)-565-3004
http://www.phassociation.org/

Pulmonary Fibrosis Foundation
230 East Ohio Street, Suite 304
Chicago, Illinois 60611-3201   1-888 733-6741
info@pulmonaryfibrosis.org

Scleroderma Foundation
300 Rosewood Drive, Suite 105
Danvers, MA 01923   (978)-463-5843
http://www.scleroderma.org

Patient Assistant Programs

ASSIST (Access Solutions and Support Team)
United Therapeutics (www.unither.com) (Adcirca®, Tyvaso®, Remodulin®)
1-877-864-8437

Boehringer Ingelheim Cares Foundation Patient Assistance
Boehringer Ingelheim (www.boehringer-ingelheim.com)
1-800-556-8317

RSVP (Revatio® Reimbursement Solution Verification Payment)
Pfizer Pharmaceuticals (www.pfizer.com)
1-888-327-RSVP (7787)

LEAP (Letairis® Education and Access Program)
Gilead Sciences (www.gilead.com)
1-866-664-LEAP (5327)

TAP (Tracleer®, Ventavis® and Opsumit® Access Program)
Actelion Pharmaceuticals (www.actelion.com)
1-866-ACTELION (228-3546)

Aim Patient Support Program (Adempas® Assistance Program)
Bayer Pharmaceuticals (www.bayer.com)
1-855-4ADEMPAS (423-3672)

Medical Information Hotline (Esbriet®)
Intermune (www.intermune.com)
1-888-486-6411

Specialty Pharmacies

Accredo (www.accredo.com)
Phone: 1-866-344-4874
Fax: 1-800-711-3526
CuraScript (www.curascript.com)
Phone: 1-866-474-8326
Fax: 1-877-305-6745
CVS/Caremark (www.caremark.com)
Phone: 1-877-242-2738
Fax: 1-877-943-1000